Diary of a
Bipolar Explorer

D1494357

Diary of a Bipolar Explorer

Lucy Newlyn

Signal Books
Oxford

First published in 2018 by
Signal Books Limited
36 Minster Road
Oxford OX4 1LY
www.signalbooks.co.uk

A catalogue record for this book is available from the British Library

ISBN 978-1-909930-63-6 Paper

Cover Design: Claire Cater
Typesetting: Tora Kelly
Cover Image: Kay Wiegand/Shutterstock
Printed in India by Imprint Press

This book is dedicated to the memory of Dr Ann McPherson (1945-2011) who was my GP for thirty years.

The GP

No nonsense from the start:
in her basement room with the green light
and a window on the garden
she saw through all excuses, pretexts, masks,
and managed to winkle confessions
from the loneliest hidden places.
Guiding me through the tunnel
she told me honestly that it would never end.

Bespectacled, girlish, tough as an ox –
she marched against the Iraq war,
talked politics in the surgery,
reminded patients that they had rights,
helped teenagers all over the world to become adults
and campaigned for assisted dying.
To have her fight your corner was to know
you could outface the playground bullies.

Humorous, relaxed, she read my poems,
liked the choughs, enjoyed our dinner at High Table.

Twenty-one years ago to this very day
when I was giving birth, she made her way
across the hospital to hold my hand.
"Just happened to be passing through,"
she said. "I thought I'd drop in to see
how you're doing..."

When she died, I was one of thousands
left nursing an immense and aching grief.
Her final legacy? The shameful hurt
of feeling thankful that she had at last
got what she wanted, a peaceful death –
even though no one could help her
to have it when she longed for it.

Contents

Introduction: The Terror of Insanity 1

Chapter One: The Showdown 9

Chapter Two: The Aftermath.. 34

Chapter Three: Crisis.. 73

Chapter Four: The Long Haul 101

Chapter Five: Retirement and Breakdown 148

Chapter Six: Re-visitings 173

Chapter Seven: Adjustment.. 195

Afterword: Bipolarity and Life-Writing 221

Select Bibliography.. 229

Acknowledgements 231

Introduction:
The Terror of Insanity

Bipolar Disorder (manic depression) involves abnormality at both ends of the mood spectrum, with swings from depression to mania which occur at variable intervals and are triggered or aggravated by external stressors.[1] Popular misconceptions about the illness are all too common. Type "Bipolar Disorder" into Google and watch amazed as a weird phantasmagoria of images unfolds before you: a brain, divided exactly down the middle – one half red, the other blue; a dead tree, the mirror image of one that's living; a woman's face as comic tragedian juggling a pair of masks; two heads joined like Janus looking before and after. There's even a gothic tinge to some of these dualities, hinting at violent tendencies: we the Bipolar Ones are seen almost as Jekyll and Hyde. The iconography puzzles me even more than the reductive labelling. Where are

---

1 In their helpful book *Bipolar Disorder The Ultimate Guide*, Sarah Owen and Amanda Saunders offer the following summary: "Bipolar disorder causes extreme mood swings that go from high and energized (manic) to low and lethargic (depressed). These swings can last from a few days to a few months." (p. 121)

the marblings, the striations? Where does red shade into blue? Where are spring and autumn in the tree's calendar? Is there no place for laughter amid tears? Give a pen to anyone who has this illness and tell them to draw it. The last thing they will think of is stark duality. Moods are not extremes which take turns; they come in multiple sounds, forms, colours; they mix, they gyrate, they layer, they shift by gradations. Why try to confine them in separate cells? Why not allow them freedom to move, to blend, and to explore? There's a whole world between the two poles. We need an open passage – or at least an accessible tunnel!

Stephen Fry, who suffers from Bipolar Disorder, is open about it. He recommends being open, to stop it from remaining the stigma that it still undoubtedly is, even in the twenty-first century. I'm now following his advice and "outing" my illness in print. As an academic who has worked for thirty-five years in Oxford University, I know that I could not have written this book until after my retirement. Professors are expected to be eccentric, but not mentally ill.

I've not been bipolar all my life, though I've always been moody. The illness set in when I was in my forties, the year my sister died and I began to write poetry. (There's a strong connection between Bipolar Disorder and creativity: Virginia Woolf, Robert Lowell, and Sylvia Plath are famous cases, all of whom suffered from a more extreme condition than mine.) Diagnosis wasn't easy in my case and it took a while before it became clear that there was a major psychiatric problem. A vigil of two sleepless nights in the hospital ward where my father lay dying triggered an episode of psychosis. I was sectioned under the Mental Health Act – a traumatic, stigmatising experience – and unable to leave hospital until fit to do so. I was in due course referred to a psychiatrist and after close monitoring under more normal circumstances I received a diagnosis.

The challenges experienced by any mother holding down a full time job are multiplied in untold ways for someone like myself with a mental illness. I've experienced the following recurring problems over the last fifteen years:

1) Paranoid delusions and visual hallucinations

2) Episodes of "hypomania" – defined as "elevation of mood leading to increased activity and energy, elation and disinhibition"[2]

---

2 "In the milder states, the patient undertakes and achieves more than usual, and is more self-confident and decisive. The patient becomes wakeful and perhaps begins new projects at night. There may be little apparent need for food. As mood elevation increases, judgement becomes impaired and activity becomes more disinhibited and tends towards grandiosity. By this stage it becomes important to protect the patient from the personally damaging consequences of the fiscal, sexual or other imprudence to which the morbid state leads." P. J. Rees & D. G. Williams *Principles of Clinical Medicine* (1995) p. 882.

3) Periods of clinical depression which have prevented me from working and participating fully in family life

4) An acute response to stress, including that caused by ordinary upheavals or minor challenges such as travel

5) Various forms of interpersonal dysfunction, at home and at work

6) Recurrent performance anxiety, especially with respect to lecturing

7) Intermittent periods of addiction – to alcohol, food, smoking, shopping, fitness regimes, email, and social media

A therapeutic approach to the illness has sometimes helped, but only in small ways. I've undergone many versions of the talking cure with skilful and sympathetic counsellors who have taught me a great deal; but the help they've given has tended to be palliative. Cognitive Behavioural Therapy isn't usually helpful for Bipolar Disorder. Mindfulness is thought to be useful, but I haven't found it so. In the day to day management of mental illness I've found GPs to be more helpful than psychiatrists, since they are not committed to any particular methodology: one just talks to them as to another human being. One GP in particular has been outstanding: I have dedicated this book to her.

Is my illness connected with lifestyle? Clinicians say that the best job for someone suffering from Bipolar Disorder is a steady one, with a regular routine and a clear framework of expectations. I can't say I've had the ideal job, then. Academic life is too unpredictable to allow patients to take proper care of themselves. At Oxford the undergraduate teaching terms last only eight weeks. Intense timetables during term-time put stress on everyone – academic and non-academic staff, as much as students. This produces a hot-house atmosphere that is good for no-one. I have managed to keep going, despite the ups and downs, because I'm lucky to have a happy marriage and a very supportive husband. I've had a successful career, greatly enjoyed my teaching, and published a number of books – including two collections of poetry of which I'm proud. My friendships have been strong, important, and most of them enduring. A lot of the time, life has been good to me, and I've had much to enjoy. I'm also immensely fortunate to have been treated by a consultant psychiatrist who's a world expert on Bipolar Disorder and I'm currently well looked after at a great psychiatric hospital which is a centre for cutting-edge research. Occasionally I'm in acute difficulties, as I was in a recent relapse which tipped me into hypomania, nearly resulting in serious psychosis. I caught the symptoms just in time: with help and the right medication I was able to pull through. I am one of the fortunate ones; others have different circumstances and more acute problems.

This book is chronological, following the shape of my life over the past fifteen years. Chapter One, *The Showdown*, provides a full and frank account of being sectioned. The rest of the book is a diary, recording the case history which followed that episode. It draws on a personal archive of medical records, emails, letters and creative writings. I have approached my experience of Bipolar Disorder from multiple perspectives – as daughter, sister, wife, mother, stepmother, friend, academic and poet. The bulk of the diary is in prose, providing a record of feelings and moods relating to my illness. It is only partly a memoir of my public life. Any references to my career are skeletal. I trace the experience of bereavement, of waiting for a diagnosis, of facing up to the implications of being diagnosed, of struggling to have my condition understood by family, colleagues and friends; and finally I explore the emotional challenges posed by retirement. Some of the diary is set in

INTRODUCTION: THE TERROR OF INSANITY

the outpatients' clinic: hospital has become a very familiar place during this period of my life. When set at home or in the workplace it tracks the day-to-day reality of depression, mania and stigma. Some of the entries take on a reflective tone similar to an essay, offering a critique of the way mental health is handled in the institutions of family and college. Short stories, embedded in the diary at appropriate chronological points, uncover acute instances of paranoia.

My experimentation with form reflects the creativity which has come out of this stressful and difficult period of life. Bipolar Disorder has benefits: I've always felt grateful for the elevated moods which have enabled me to keep writing. I have occasionally used poetry as well as prose to illuminate what it feels like to be bipolar. Poetry is an essential tool – not just because I'm a poet, but because this particular medium is closely allied to my illness and a by-product of it. Formal experimentation on the boundary between poetry and prose is also important to the kind of narrative I need to present. To be true to life my writing must acknowledge the in-between and mixed states of mood disorder. The mental condition I describe does not accommodate itself to the normal tidy distinctions between forms, and no straightforward narrative mode will do.

DIARY OF A BIPOLAR EXPLORER

There are numerous books on Bipolar Disorder and bereavement; I provide a selective reading-list on the final page of this book. My diary adds to the wealth of material that already exists – not as a guide or a handbook, but as one patient's account of what it is to be bipolar. My title, *Diary of a Bipolar Explorer*, draws attention to formal experimentation as well as to the adventures of mental process and discovery. I hope that by demystifying Bipolar Disorder I will help others in overcoming the stigma and engaging creatively with the struggle. Above all else, I hope this book will do something to diminish the terror of insanity.

Chapter One:
The Showdown

To be a comprehensive account – telling the truth, the whole truth, and nothing but the truth – my story would have to begin sixty years ago in my birth-place, Kampala. But even such a long narrative would be highly selective. This one starts in September 2002, when my dad was dying. His was not the only death that was on the minds of those who gathered round him that night; my older sister Sally had died two years earlier...

The Competition

The call came. We must get to Leeds as quickly as possible. There was panic, phoning round among family members and some despair at discovering that no trains would get us there that night. We decided the best plan was to drive to Bristol, pick up Gill and Kate (my two surviving sisters) and head up North. I packed an overnight bag and got in the car. It was a long roundabout journey from Oxford to Leeds. My husband Martin drove but I got no sleep, an omission for which I would in due course pay heavily.

We reached Leeds at 3.00 a.m on the Tuesday. The hospital – St James's, known familiarly as Jimmie's – was deathly quiet like a morgue, except for the brightness of the lighting. None of us had dared to phone in advance to discover if dad was alive or dead, so we arrived at the ward very tense. I remember the relief we all felt as we looked in and found him still breathing with mum alongside him. He was very thin and extremely frail – more so than when I had seen him a few days earlier. There was a black bruise on his bony hand where the needle of the drip entered a vein. He couldn't speak and he wore an oxygen-mask that slipped from his face, needing constant re-adjustment. Martin stayed a while before heading back to Oxford. He was missed almost the moment he had gone. Mum, shattered by long anxiety, went off home to her flat to get about eight hours of much-needed sleep.

Gill, Kate and I were left prop-less, clustered round our father's death-bed. The scene was a cross between a Victorian melodrama and bad-taste derivative tragedy. Were we the three sisters in *King Lear*, or perhaps in Chekhov? It hardly matters which: we all knew that the one daughter my dad would have most loved to see was nowhere to be seen – two years dead, no earthly help to anyone. (The only time I ever saw my father cry was in the lead-up to Sally's death.)

We began comparing notes – talking in whispers at first, wondering if what we kept seeing in dad was a smile of recognition, or just the effect of medication. Something told me that mum's urgent phone-call had been a false alarm. I had watched Sally die in her early forties, and I knew that even the very old, even the very sick, take a long time to let go: there's always a great deal of waiting.

Soon we were competing as usual – each to be the one to notice our dad's needs most intuitively and to look after him the best. We felt he wasn't getting the attention he deserved. We didn't understand how the drip worked, so our concern centred on the oxygen-mask: being the first to spot that it had slipped, being the quickest and the most adept at adjusting it.

Dad was unconscious most of the time and his breathing was shallow. A kind friendly nurse with a broad Leeds accent kept popping her head round the door. She said we had a lovely dad; that his eyes were attractive. He did habitually have a very surprised and intelligent look, accentuated under these conditions. He reminded me of Sally. In her last days Sally became gaunt because of the cancer. Her face became dad's. Now the reverse process was taking place. Looking at his head propped on the pillow I kept thinking it was hers.

By mid-morning I was very tired, having been awake since 8.00 a.m on Monday. But I was too overwrought to try taking a nap somewhere in the hospital. When mum dropped in at 11.00 a.m. to relieve us, we recognised that we had a long watch ahead, that a rota for watching would be needed. We three sisters went back to mum's flat, leaving her to some quiet time with dad. During the next six hours, I was so anxious I couldn't have slept even if I had tried.

We got a taxi back to the hospital at about 4.00 p.m. When we arrived on the ward, mum was cheerful, but we already felt that the rota was not going to work. Because Gill was feeling very unwell she and mum went back to the flat and I stayed in the ward with Kate. The others came back at supper time to relieve us. As our collective anxiety mounted I suggested that I would join Gill and Kate at the pub for a drink. At the pub, did we eat anything? I don't remember doing so and there is no record of a meal in the notes I made shortly after the events of that night. I drank a half of Guinness; we continued joking. The mood felt all wrong. I explained that there'd been too much alcohol in my life since Sally's death: right now it wasn't what I needed. I said good-night and went back to dad.

At the hospital Mum was given a little side-ward to sleep in. It would have been very sensible for me to take a nap too, but I felt I really didn't want to let up on watching because dad might suddenly take a turn for the worse. I had now been constantly awake since Monday morning. Mum went home around 3.00 a.m. At last I had him completely to myself.

The vigil

It was so very quiet on the ward. Sometimes a nurse came in to check how dad was doing; but otherwise I kept my vigil more or less without interruption. I was able now and again to read short passages from Susan Hill's *Strange Meeting*. I'd been reading a lot about the First World War since Sally died. I wanted to understand survivor's guilt. The massive scale of suffering in the trenches had been helping me to get my own grief in perspective. I was gripped by Hill's study of two men whose temperaments are opposite: Hilliard repressed and emotionally stifled, Barton open, affectionate, frank, generous. I felt this book had something very powerful to communicate. Despite the terrible context of the war it showed the melting of reserve in a cold person. A few days earlier, under an apple tree at home, I had sat weeping because the book moved me so much; now here I was on dad's ward, with only pages to go before the ending...

> In the night, he woke and heard the guns and his heart thudded, and he sat up and said aloud, 'Jesus God, don't let him be killed, don't let him be killed.' And did not mind that Barton might have awoken and heard him. 'Don't let him be killed'.

It was time for Lights Out on the ward, but in the white corridors the strip-lights were glaring so brightly that their clarity hurt. The hours passed slowly. I lost all sense of chronology in this busy place where the night-nurses worked so hard. I began to observe them closely, curious about their work and why they enjoyed it so much. They were excellent at keeping each other's spirits up, at jollying me along, and at talking with dad. I felt ashamed not to have realised how much could be communicated by and to a dying person. The professionals had skills I could learn from; they made direct eye contact with dad whenever possible and they kept squeezing his hand. Gradually, as the night wore on, I began to imitate them and to learn their approach to the process of dying. I felt that what was happening to me was momentous, and that I must write it down while I was experiencing it. In between scribbling in the back of *Strange Meeting* my focus was still on dad's oxygen-mask, which now and again I adjusted. As time wore on it morphed in my mind into a gas-mask, and I seemed to see my father lying in a trench on the Somme. My grandfather died in the First World War; my dad fought in the Second, having never known his father. Two time-schemes became muddled, blurring two separate identities.

In the back of *Strange Meeting* I made my notes; and the shape of my thoughts was determined by the content of the novel – by Hilliard and Barton, whose contrasting temperaments seemed to hover over everything that was happening to me. Descriptions of conditions in the trenches began to seep into the way I saw the scenes around me in this Spartan hospital ward where NHS cuts were taking their toll:

The trench was quite deep, cut into the chalk, and at the beginning the sandbags had been removed and the parapets built up again. But as they went further on, work had ceased, the floor was a mess of rubble, the sides broken. Pit props, shovels and bales of wire cluttered every traverse, and the duckboards, laid in preparation for the coming winter, and the wet weather, were often broken or rotted away.

I felt I had something to communicate about how war could be stopped. I was convinced there would be no further World Wars if soldiers could be better cared for. I wanted to tell the world that when people are sick and dying they need to have physical contact and to be talked to authentically. The Northern voices of the team on dad's ward seemed so healing, and they laughed and hugged and joked. Their humour held them together, whereas our dysfunctional family team was a failure. I wanted to shout out about the stupidity of using oxygen-masks that looked like First World War gas-masks. All ugly things should be removed from the wards. There should be colour, texture, light, movement, growth. If the hospitals were more beautiful there would be a better chance that the sick would survive. I took a walk around to see if I could find an available nurse – and everywhere, in all the wards, I saw people of all ages lying in trenches with or without gas-masks: they were the sick, the wounded, and the dying.

As they rounded the next corner walking towards the spot from which the cry for stretcher bearers had just gone up, they came upon a blockage in the trench-way, a mess of burnt sandbags and earth, shrapnel and mutilated bodies…

Where had the nurses gone? There weren't enough of them.

From this point onward I was disturbed by extremely powerful feelings. I can remember addressing the Matron in tones of urgency. If enough help could be found, if these sick people could be saved, perhaps the next war could be averted. She took me into her office. How flat her voice sounded as she ran through a few pat phrases: "everyone gets overwrought in situations like this. We are concerned." She lacked warmth, she was too professional. By contrast, I was a prophet who could save the world. I had seen for the first time the secret of the universe. I had been admitted to a band of comrades whose message was love and peace. It was like returning to infancy and seeing nothing but goodness in my parents. I told a few more people about this loudly. One of the night-nurses asked me when I had last slept and looked alarmed when I gave my answer. "Go and sit in that chair and get some sleep immediately," he commanded. I ignored him, and found another night-nurse with whom I felt a bond, which I expressed openly. I felt that this nurse (let's call him David) had elected me as a member of the band of special people.

Diary of a Bipolar Explorer

I went up to the receptionist to check with her that what I believed to be my initiation or "baptism" had actually taken place. She told me I had made some very disturbing remarks to David. Soon afterwards, mum came with Gill and Kate to relieve me from my watch. It was Gill's turn to be alongside dad.

Trial and Final Judgment

It was Wednesday morning. I had done something wrong on the ward and was now under pressure to return to my mum's flat. I felt I was undergoing a trial. My "crime" was not my behaviour on the ward, it was nothing less than patricide. I had been framed by my sisters.

Gill and Kate were guilty. They had gone away and left me on my own in the hospital. I was innocent, but I was being tried for dad's murder. I understood that he had received an injection to put him to sleep for ever; they had wanted this to happen, and had arrived in the hospital to ensure that I was not there to protect him. I knew for sure that they were disguising their lack of love. When I first started shouting, it was to tell everyone that they were not carers. There were only a few of us who truly understood how suffering could be averted. I was their leader.

Chapter One: The Showdown

Somehow I was removed from the hospital and into my mum's car. I can recall feeling angry with Kate for engineering my removal. She was not in the "clan". I felt she did not know about love. I kept pointing at mum and saying, "She's the carer." I'm unable to reconstruct the next part of what happened except through memories that have been recounted to me much later, after long silence, by Kate and by mum. Their accounts differ sharply in several respects; at the end of this book I have gone into the differences. After all these years I'm still disturbed and frightened by my own memory lapse and the loss of continuity in myself that it entails.

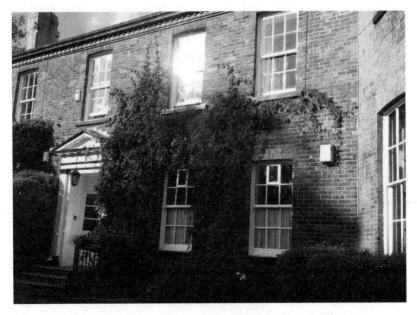

The threshold to my mother's flat, at 'The Elms' in Chapel Allerton

DIARY OF A BIPOLAR EXPLORER

The one thing we can all agree on is that I hugged mum very hard, saying, "You're the one, the only one." (She was the best of the Very Good People, the chosen one who could help to avert all coming evils.) Mum was so frightened by the strength of the hug that Kate took a quick decision to pull me forcibly away from her by my hair and sit on me to prevent my moving. She then dialled 999. Mum said to the receptionist on the phone: "We have an hysteric" and gave confirmation that violence was involved, thus instigating the arrival of a police car as well as an ambulance. The siren was harsh – something between a scream and a melancholy wail. The police quickly established that I had *not* been violent and that they were not needed, so they disappeared from the scene. A kind paramedic coaxed me inside the house where we talked for a while. He persuaded me to get into the ambulance. I can remember lots of questions, the voice of Kate in front, and a sense of persecution. We arrived at Casualty and Kate talked to a Consultant, who explained to her that I must be sectioned. There were two guards outside the room where I was incarcerated. She signed the official form with a trembling hand.

Two narratives of my own blur and intermingle from the moment of entering the back of the ambulance. In the

CHAPTER ONE: THE SHOWDOWN

first, I was being taken to Casualty, which in my hallucinating brain became a "Special Unit". This had been set up to put family members through a series of tests in which their authenticity as carers would be assessed. It was also a unit for the reception and recording of Communal Memory, to which only members of the Very Good had access, and only after their "baptism". I was being transferred to the Special Unit by virtue of my endurance and empathy. I had just been "baptised" and this had given me access to some secret information which needed to be imparted to the world. My memory would supply a long list of Jews whose identities had been lost, together with the addresses of the slaughter-houses in which they had been expunged from memory. It was believed by everyone in the Special Unit that I had *special powers of memory*, and that when I had imparted my knowledge, not only would many families recover their lost identities, but there would be no Second or Third World Wars. I would be recognised as the Healing Prophet I truly was. My special status would be celebrated in a big World Wide Programme. I was being carried to a Press Conference: I would communicate my message to the world; the world would listen; the world would be saved and healed.

The second narrative was very different, yet it seemed to be inextricable from the first. I realise now that it must have been prompted by the brief appearance of a police car outside my mum's flat. In this scenario I knew for certain by the loud wailing siren that I had been arrested and was being carried to my trial. The Special Unit would be investigating which members of my family were the real carers. Of course I had been wrongly accused; I hoped my authenticity would be revealed and my sisters exposed. But I was terrified by the possibility that I would be found wanting.

Arriving in Casualty I thought I had been put in prison. When a psychiatrist interviewed me I didn't know who I was or even what time of day it was. I had turned into a strange thing I couldn't recognise as myself. I sat on a seat which was also a toilet in a large white empty room on my own where a strong bright light shone on me perpetually. I shouted for a long, long time. When I was let out of the observation room I saw the A&E area, where people were lying on stretchers or trolleys. I was sure they were war-victims; there was one whose face was bloated – her whole body was swollen and it seemed to be in a sack. She looked like my mum. There were other people whose heads I could see over the tops of screens, and I thought two of them were my sisters. I kept hearing their voices, and they seemed to be lying about me – their accounts of me were a tissue of lies, designed to show that I was no carer. They wanted me punished. I kept screaming at the top of my voice: "LISTEN".

I had patches of lucidity in which I thought I was going to be rewarded and praised for staying as long as I did with dad – as if I had won First Prize for an endurance test. I was interrogated by many people. Most were coldly anonymous but some had friendly open faces and I felt they were on my side. I was terrified by a man with big black boots and leather gloves who resembled a member of the Gestapo. I asked him if I was innocent or guilty, shouting out that I was due to be publicly shamed. In among all the screaming I can remember going through violent jerking movements with my arms, my head, and my facial muscles. Someone arrived and asked me to confirm my name and my address. I saw the bloated face of my mum again and she seemed to be evil. I know for a fact that there were no objects I could hurl around – the room was empty. Yet I'm sure I hurled something; it feels even now as if I did. Then came the patterned curtains and Martin's face between them, smiling. He had received an urgent phone-call and driven all the way back to Leeds but it wasn't his face I saw: he looked sinister at the same time as kind and although his eyes had deep sockets they were also a flat motif in the curtain's patterning. He seemed to have something growing out of the side of his face; he looked like a dying soldier.

Martin tells me he was with me as I was transferred by ambulance from a cubicle in Casualty to a quiet room in the hospital's Psychiatric Wing not far from my father's ward. When I arrived there, the two narratives of Trial and Press Conference were still going on in my head. Martin was leading me to a television studio where the cameras were ready for the reception of my World Wide Message. But outside the ward was a big black bin labelled DOMESTIC WASTE ONLY. I was a lunatic. I would end up in that bin.

Safe inside the Psychiatric Wing I was still hallucinating: two of the staff seemed alternately my friends and my enemies. I liked their faces but couldn't trust them. I thought everything would all come clear immediately and that the trial would end, but it didn't. I was so terrified that I begged forgiveness for my crimes again and again. Some time passed, but that is now trackless. I remember a crowded room, where several rows of doctors stared at me taking their notes. I sensed then that I was facing a panel of judges. I knew myself to be a prophet and believed myself to be present at the Final Judgment to give my testimony.

Chapter One: The Showdown

Someone – I have no recollection of his face or name – summed up the evidence against me. My voice was for justice and everlasting peace, but I was judged unworthy. After that I can remember only a feeling of monumental let-down and a sense of shame. Sleep at last came.

Apologies

After the Final Judgment I slept the sleep of the just in a solitary ward, watched by an eye in the door. Did they think I'd be using the sheets and two pillowcases tied together to hang myself from the ceiling? Did they think I'd be trying to climb out of there? On the third day, rested, I saw where I was and who they were – even perhaps who I was. I can't recall if the sun shone; only that everything seemed very connected and very clear. They let me out for an hour (accompanied, of course) to visit my dad – and to make my apologies to the staff in the ward where he lay dying.

My gaoler was Norah. She smoked a lot and had long red shiny nails which she kept filing. She sustained a running commentary on life, making me laugh. We walked together into the open air... then indoors again, along the terrible white corridors. The wards looked different in the light of day. Everywhere, lying in their beds, I saw the sick and the dying – but the trenches had gone, this was no longer the Somme. Wheeling trolleys to and fro the nurses and the doctors were on their rounds. There were house-plants, flowers, cards, and chocolate boxes at bedsides. Patients shouted greetings to each other across the wards; visitors were coming and going.

The Matron on my dad's ward heard what I had to say: I was sorry that I had behaved so strangely – would she convey my apologies to everyone on the ward? She frowned and shook her head, muttering something about how sleep was necessary; that what I'd said that night wasn't tolerable. I hurried away with Norah.

Dad's white face peeked over the bedclothes. A cradle of wires held him gently, like a child born before anyone was ready. His eyes were a long way back in their sockets and they were wakeful. He was so weak he could scarcely move his arms. His hands were skinny and the veins stood up like dark wandering ridges. He still wore that oxygen-mask which kept slipping.

I was shy and had too much to say; my voice was hoarse and painful after all the shouting. So I kept silent, biding my time. Norah was loquacious: she gave us a digest of the world news, interspersed with acid commentary. Then I read Binyon's "The Burning of the Leaves" aloud, thinking of Grove Lane, and how dad always loved autumn fires:

CHAPTER ONE: THE SHOWDOWN

All the spices of June are a bitter reek,
All the extravagant riches spent and mean.
All burns! The reddest rose is a ghost;
Sparks whirl up, to expire in the mist: the wild
Fingers of fire are making corruption clean.

He lay there quietly, with listening eyes. Norah patted him gently and said that we must go.

In the lift I asked if she thought he'd recognised me. "Sorry," she answered. "I don't know. We can come back tomorrow." We went the next day and the day after and the day after that – she collected me, carrying her copy of *The Guardian*. Together we selected the best bits for him to hear. I told Norah about dad's work in Africa. I think she liked our visits – she took a shine to my dad and said that he was "hanging on in there like a trooper". She had a loud Leeds voice and a laugh that crackled like Binyon's fire. Her critique of the world was devastating.

As a patient sectioned under the Mental Health Act, classified as a danger to myself and others, I was still a prisoner in the Psychiatric Wing, where it would soon be necessary to prove to my gaolers that I was well enough to go home. I was summoned for a meeting with them twice, and they informed me that David (the nurse on the ward whom I had offended with my remarks) had decided not to press charges – a kindness for which I'm grateful to this day. The doctors gave me more information about what had happened to the chemicals in my body as a result of being sleep-deprived. They also advised me that I had undergone withdrawal symptoms after doing without alcohol for three days: this indicated that I must cut down on alcohol in future. They informed me that because of this psychotic episode I would be referred to a psychiatrist on returning home: they were concerned about the pattern of ill health that had followed my sister's death. I didn't like them much – when I met them, they were arranged in serried ranks, looking accusatory. I talked to them, but less freely than to the nurses.

I had soon become accustomed to the shabby Victorian house in which they looked after me and the others. I liked the communal meals, but the eye in the door was extremely irksome. I had no privacy. Although the doctors were aloof and stern, the nurses were kind like the ones on my dad's ward. They had an aura. My birthday went past while I was there; I don't remember celebrating it. But Martin drove from Oxford to see me on several occasions, bringing clothes and books – and messages from my daughter Emma, whom I was missing keenly. My sister Kate was advised not to come and my mum never came — she wanted to avoid visits at a time that was so difficult. This is what I wrote in my notebook after the fierce resentment at my loss of liberty had worn off:

I feel safe here and my room is so comfortable and nice. I can look through into a little nursery connected to my room, with a cot in it and lots of lovely things for children. Emma would love the nursery so much. The staff are kind and I feel very serene and reassured. I would like to stay here for a bit longer. I've got to know all the patients individually and I'll write about them another time...

After a while I was allowed out on my own to see my father for much longer. I would sit for hours reading to him from an anthology of poems. It wasn't that I was sure he could hear me, though I think he sometimes did. It was just good to sit in quiet with the window open, watching him sleeping or awake and not have to say much — just to hear the rhythms of the poems, sounds on the ward, and traffic noise from the street below. There were long peaceful silences. The nurses sometimes came in to check his drip or change his bed. They greeted us cheerily and always patted his arm affectionately. One of them was

Jamaican. She said "bless" a lot: her voice rose and fell like music.

One day I read him this poem by Edward Thomas:

Sowing

It was a perfect day
For sowing; just
As sweet and dry was the ground
As tobacco-dust.

I tasted deep the hour
Between the far
Owl's chuckling first soft cry
And the first star.

A long stretched hour it was;
Nothing undone
Remained; the early seeds
All safely sown.

And now, hark at the rain,
Windless and light,
Half a kiss, half a tear,
Saying good-night.

CHAPTER ONE: THE SHOWDOWN

On that one occasion I'm convinced he heard. His eyes were wide open. He smiled and squeezed my hand. That wasn't the last time I saw him, but can I be allowed the tender fiction that it was? It would make better sense of things. Soon afterwards I was discharged from hospital and never saw him again. I'm sorry I wasn't with him when he died. I'm sorry he didn't see the next spring. I'm sorry I never got to go back with him to Kampala.

Reflections on this episode

My psychosis in Leeds was without question the most frightening, traumatic experience of my life. It would eventually lead to my diagnosis of Bipolar Disorder. I don't regard the diagnosis in any way as a blessing; but at least it put me in touch with the psychiatrists who look after me now. A more direct outcome of the psychotic episode was my decision to give up alcohol – something I succeeded in doing for ten years, without difficulty after the first few weeks. One of the lasting negative outcomes has been the stigma of having been sectioned. Another, which became clear with the passage of time, is that my experiences that morning left me with PTSD (Post-Traumatic Stress Disorder), the main stressors being as follows: ambulance sirens, very bright lights, the sign "DOMESTIC WASTE

ONLY" and the threshold of my mother's flat in Leeds. The most painful of these, with damaging repercussions for me and my whole family, is the threshold.

In the notes that I made immediately afterwards (while still at the Psychiatric Wing) I find this gloss on what caused the psychosis:

> *I was desperate to sleep but reluctant to leave the ward because I wanted to stay with dad. I wanted the ultimate test of endurance. I wanted to win the competition with my sisters for dad's love, and I wanted to find out what it looked like as he died, as well as to discover if I felt better afterwards than I had after Sally's death.*

Looking back fifteen years after the episode, I read this as a painful but illuminating way of understanding what happened. Winning the test of endurance was, for me, a means of compensating for having failed to be in the same room as Sally when she died. I had been downstairs in her kitchen making tea.

It's significant that for fifteen years following the episode in Leeds my family never once had a general discussion about what happened and that it was never mentioned to me by my mother during that time. It has had the status of a taboo – a taboo that has only just been broken as I write this book. I think that the sense of stigma I've felt in relation to my subsequent diagnosis of Bipolar Disorder has its origins in the shame surrounding my having been sectioned; though of course there are wider than family reasons for feeling stigmatised – as I would in due course discover.

Finally, a word on the narrative that I have written here. Its true heroes are not my dysfunctional family – we were all too distraught to look after each other. Nor are they the clan of the Very Good, who dominated my hallucinations throughout the psychosis. No, the only heroes here are the underpaid nurses on my father's ward who looked after dad so well and the tremendous people who cared for me in the Psychiatric Wing, restoring me to balance. When I left the hospital after two weeks under their care, I felt I had made some friends for life. Thanks most of all to Norah, who was a chum, a superlative professional, and a *mensch*.

Chapter Two:
The Aftermath

I've returned to Oxford. Dad is nearer to death with every day. I hear about this from mum only on the phone and feel strangely disconnected. My doctor has told me to stay away from the place where the psychosis happened, even at the cost of never seeing dad again. I don't talk about the psychotic episode with mum; she never raises the subject – do I feel lost to her? If so, how strange, because I'm still here, I'm still her daughter. I go over and over the events of that morning in Leeds but feel calmer. Abstinence from alcohol is making my life more coherent. I'm medicated, steady, seeing my doctor regularly for advice. It's still the summer vacation. The trees in our garden are heavy with apples, which I pick during the day and bake into apple-cakes and crumbles. I make soup and bread; I clear the kitchen, repaint the shelves in the larder. When I walk with Emma to school I feel whole, I feel clean, I feel grounded.

Now I'm at the fairground in St Giles, an annual Oxford festivity. I'm watching Emma go round and round on a horse which rises and falls slowly. Her thumb's in her mouth; with the other hand she waves at me. There's a loud noise all around us: music, shouting, laughter, and a high-pitched wailing siren. The sound pierces me. I'm back at my mum's threshold, the day of the psychosis. Panic wells up; I lose eye-contact with Emma.

I'm standing outside Emma's school, waiting to collect her. (I think of my own mum, waiting to collect me when I was her age.) All the mothers are there, looking clean and whole and grounded. Theirs is a club to which I can't belong. They speak of what they'll do when they get home —what they'll cook for supper. I think of Sally's death, my dad in hospital, and being shut away in the psychiatric ward. They speak and all I hear is nothingness. I see their mouths opening, shutting; I see Emma coming out of school. She doesn't wave; she looks uncomfortable. I shuffle away from all the mothers. This is what grief is. A blankness. I wonder what they think of me. I wonder how much they know.

October 2002: Telling the truth

He died today, so Emma must be told. She's only six. Sally died when she was four, when she was too young to understand. Now far too old for swings and roundabouts, we go straight home. I sit her on my knee. Calm at first, she knows death to be something not altogether strange or new. Then comes the moment I have not prepared. "What happens afterwards?" "Nothing." I've never seen a human being stare so long, with eyes so bleak and bare. I hold her as the hugeness of the fact sweeps through her and she clings to me pleading: "No, mum. It can't end with nothing." She's wracked, and I am too.

Her first flinching over, she's brave and makes her peace with grandpa's death. I'm glad I haven't lied, or stopped her flow of curiosity with mention of a grave. When asked I've let her clearly know where his ashes will go after he's burned. What would have happened if I'd waffled instead – told her some feeble fiction, or in cowardice compared him to a cloud or rain, not dead but translated? Would she have shared my longing – or resisted, scared?

October 2002: The funeral

I'm mostly numb. Standing at the threshold to mum's house I can hear the siren; I can see a bright white light shining directly into my face and involuntarily I picture the eye in the door at the Psychiatric Wing. I hear people talking. I see them opening and shutting their mouths. Most of what they say is inaudible to me; my thoughts are racing and I'm disconnected. At the funeral there's only a small group of family and a couple of my mum's dearest friends. Seeing Gill and Kate again I feel vulnerable. We each say something at the short service. I read one of my poems. As we leave the room, we all touch the wicker coffin in which dad lies. I imagine him inside it, small and frail.

December 2002: The memorial celebration

We leave Emma behind and drive North, those terrible miles again, each one closer to the scene of dying. We convene at the West Yorkshire Playhouse with a large gathering of old friends. I'm in a trance; my main preoccupation is how to get through the event, how to hold myself together as I pay public tribute and read my poem to this group of theatre lovers. The scene is theatrical, the stress immense. But it's less bad than when I did the same thing after Sally's death: this is a celebration of a long, very fulfilled life – not a funeral for one that was tragically curtailed. I'm like a performing animal, separate from my emotions: the oldest surviving daughter, the one who's experienced at public speaking. I feel raw and exposed. My mouth is dry, I sweat. Only when the music starts do I understand how deep the feelings go.

Diary of a Bipolar Explorer

There was never any question of choosing another song. This one, only this one, would carry us along, its searing truth a kind of secular family gospel:

> Close the coalhouse door, lad
> There's blood inside
> Blood from broken hands and feet
> Blood that's dried on pit-black meat
> Blood from hearts that know no beat
> Close the coalhouse door, lad,
> There's blood inside...

Dad's life is in these words: his compassion, his politics, and his early research into mining. Alex Glasgow was his friend, and his singing touches us all. When we play the recording, it's as if a disused mine has opened. The pain of centuries rises up from underground so that everyone can feel it, touch it, breathe it. If dad were here, he'd know that our song was chosen well.

January 2003: Return to work

The days are cold and dark and bare. Hilary Term has begun. Two new colleagues have been holding the fort at work during my sick leave. I threw myself into Admissions just before Christmas and I've now resumed my full role in College. My concern for students with mental health problems has intensified after my psychotic episode. I feel vulnerable and scared. It'll be hard to keep balanced as the pace of term increases.

February 2003: Protest in London

Hundreds of thousands of people converge on London to protest against the invasion of Iraq. I'm agonised by the prospect of war and caught up in the wave of anger against Tony Blair, but too depressed to join the march. I hunker down with Emma and Martin at home. Turning on the news, who do I see but my own GP Ann McPherson, caught on camera among the marching protesters? What energy and force of character to be there! I kick myself for not going but I'm marching alongside her in spirit.

April 2003: Play

There's no shortage of photos in Emma's first three years: a lively child, often pictured in the garden under our cherry-tree. She's used to a camera and smiling brightly. Then suddenly they come to a stop: in the last one she stands awkward and unsettled beside a Christmas tree –

something doll-like in the way she looks at me. That was the week that Sally died. No photos have since been taken. The albums are hidden away.

I can't play with her. No matter how hard I try, I can't leave my work behind. I *cannot* play.

I spend lavishly on her, buying her all that I can buy. She has the entire range of Sylvanians, little forest creatures who wear elaborately human clothes and go to school and are raised in families. They fill her room; she needs them all and plays with them every day. I can't even muster the energy to watch her play.

I go to London with her to avoid the men who come to fell the cherry-tree. We get lost in the underground because I can't stay to read the signs or find the way. When we get home at last it's nearly dark. There's an absence in our back garden which fills the sky. There's a hole in the lawn where there used to be a tree. We stand in silence. There's nothing we can say. She's silent all evening – and she cannot play.

May 2003: Creativity

Where has it come from, this energy to write, this focus on writing? I'm not well, I don't feel balanced, yet each day when I sit down at my desk a new poem comes into being. I write about my childhood. Although I don't write directly about dad or Sally yet the places that fill my poems are connected with them. The house and garden in Headingley, the streets surrounding the house – I can picture them all distinctly. I grieve for the loss of childhood; I memorialise people by writing an elegy for a lost place.

My focus is immense; I can concentrate all day, sometimes well into the night too. My brain feels sharp; I don't seem to need much sleep. I finish a poem one day, revise it the next and then on the third day when I wake a new one is already forming. They all connect: one leads directly and inevitably to the next, like a system of ginnels. I have a whole sequence clearly in mind. I'm constrained by the limitations of time and space in which I live, yet in poetry I find a clearing, I break free.

June 2003: Workshops

Together with fellow-poet Jenny Lewis I'm running creative writing workshops for my students at St Edmund Hall. We have a grant to cover the costs of a book we're putting together. We're tracking the benefits of creative writing in an academic context. The work is exciting, liberating. To be with these students as they discover their voices as writers is one of the most fulfilling experiences in my career. I feel weirdly released; the workshops give me a high like walking in the sun and wind. I'm off balance; creativity feels dangerous and exhilarating.

October 2003: An ordinary day

It's a mood, the place from which I move only to make weak tea. Its official name is almost as drab as the sofa where it sits me. The sofa's drabness is in it and the turning-grey cushions have only it as their fabric. Boring as boredom, for weeks now it has clung around me like an odour. It has known me for so long we're more or less identical twins. Inside my pores it got a long time ago and ordinary stale it is. My body wears it round me like cladding; I am what it wears, and immovably solid. Even if I turn the people to face me going up and down the street they move only with it. I watch for it to turn me; I can remember it turning. Meanwhile it sits and I won't name it.

November 2003: The library

It's no use on a morning like this – the serried spines on the shelves repel. I can't even open the five books I ordered, which line the desk in disapproval. There's a tunnel that goes back thirty years from this desk to the same one thirty years ago. If I stay very still I can hear the familiar sound of feet passing, the shuffle of papers, coughing.

It's hard to tell how many people are really reading. They could just be sitting, turning the pages. Not much has changed in the tunnel. It will be there still at 5.30. It will be there still at 5.30. It will be there at 5.30 still.

December 2003: The waiting-room

The designers must have given thought to this. Perhaps they think in terms of allegory. Upright chairs, mostly empty. No pot-plants. Nothing on the walls. No table piled with magazines as there would be at the dentist's, the doctor's, the hairdresser's. Nothing in the middle but an area of floor – to be walked round, occasionally crossed. If someone comes in and sits down you can't look at them, you have to look at the middle. If you're in the mood for it, that's where you find the nub of the allegory: that bland area in the middle, with nothing in it, is "Normality" – a social construct. As the hands of the clock inch round, all you can do is watch the middle while the edges look away.

Diary of a Bipolar Explorer

January 2004: Whatever it is...

In a house, at the turn of a landing-place
before going upstairs or down

in a garden at the edge of a tree's shadow
or at a threshold, when the door's left slightly ajar

on a street at night where the kerb is lit up
then hidden, and footfalls are fading.

It has no colour, texture, scent, or sound
so you'd expect it to slip away, but still

it sticks around – especially at airports
in the long wait after checking in.

Is it a medium in which I move,
or something outside myself that I feel and see?

It clings to me like a miasma;
it dogs my days like anger, envy, shame.

I could pass it on if it were less pervasive.
I could shuffle it off, if it only had a name.

CHAPTER TWO: THE AFTERMATH

February 2004: The tipping-point

They tell me what they think it is before discharging me and advising me to inform College. They say there's no known cure for Bipolar Disorder. The pattern of my illness seems to be one of long drawn-out anxiety and depression – for which I can take medication – overlaid by sporadic highs. They recommend a Seasonal Affective Disorder Lamp to counteract the low mood that often accompanies light deficiency. There's no question of going on lithium as things stand at present, though it's an option if I have a relapse. They say that it's a good idea to tell a colleague about my condition, so that this person can watch out for the beginnings of manic or depressive episodes and their effects on my performance at work. I'll tell my closest colleague – though there's scarcely any need, as Martin is a Fellow of the same college.

They say I mustn't see Bipolar Disorder as a stigma; more as a condition – something I'm to carry with me always. They tell me it's been there for a long time – possibly all my life, but latent, with a tipping-point at some time after Sally died. A tipping-point, they emphasise, is not an origin or cause. I think in visual metaphors; "tipping-point" is a vivid one. The first thing I picture is Emma on a see-saw, going up, going down, her excited face small and clear: my strong legs controlling the momentum, her feet on tip-toes as she touches the ground, her rising voice letting out a sound – or us both letting one out together, is it yelp or sigh? Then Emma again playing with the kitchen scales: lips pursed, eyes intent, practising the removal of one gram, two grams, three, four, five... till one side of the scales rises slowly and the other falls. And then again, watching something she should not have pushed, something that teeters; her frightened eyes as she sees it lean to make a swift inevitable arc through the air, then the shattering sound as it hits the ground.

"Is the condition genetic?" I ask, picturing my mother's lifelong energy, my father in his retirement, withdrawn. They give some kind of answer, vague and unsatisfactory. I scarcely listen; I'm beside myself with fear. As I get up to leave, lugging my diagnosis, I'm picturing Emma again – the years passing, the years to come; and the tipping-point for her. Again, my daughter's face at the end of the see-saw, small and clear.

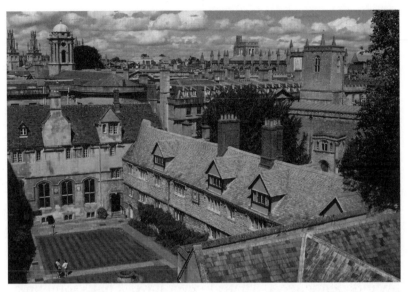

The front quad of St Edmund Hall from above (photo by Christopher Cornwell)

Spring 2004: College and family

How does my family fit into the patterns of my relationships at work? Why is it that my work has become so all-consuming? Is my situation complicated by the fact that I have a husband who works in the same College as me, so that we never really get away from our work, carrying College-related issues home with us and never switching off? I'm hyperactive in College. I throw myself into my teaching; I take on more additional jobs (pastoral and extra-curricular) than I should. My students are like my children; I focus almost all my energy on their lives and needs. Even when I'm low-spirited this contact with young people feels worthwhile. In all this, there's an undertow of sadness. Why can't I find the same energies and skills where my own daughter is concerned? Is there a competition between her and my students for attention? Does she feel resentful that they take so much of my time?

When Emma was born I was shocked, the first night, to find myself alone with her – she was crying so often and needing milk every hour or so. I felt like a drip-feed machine. It took months to come to terms with the loss of my independence; perhaps I never have. That's sometimes how it feels with the undergraduates in my care, within a collegiate university that prides itself on the tutorial system. Every one of my students, negotiating the difficult passage to maturity, is vulnerable. I watch their struggles to succeed in an institution where academic success is paramount, but where they're also required to be social animals in a partying culture. I observe them undergoing personal problems which feed into their work; the pretence that these can be separated from their work makes no sense. The university and college have pastoral duties and there are various structures in place to support undergraduates – but these can seem inadequate or perfunctory; often the students are wary and unwilling to ask for help. There's a large-scale conspiracy of silence surrounding the appalling loneliness that mental health problems can induce in young people who are dedicating themselves to intellectual endeavour. Women students often suffer the effects of institutional blindness more than men and are drawn more actively into supporting each other. To function well as families, reforms in colleges are needed.

In all this I observe that my own involvement in reform runs alongside the problems I myself experience. Like anyone who takes an active interest in the pastoral life of a college I need to stand back, to be less involved. My college feels *too much* like a family.

Summer 2004: A breakthrough

Hurrah! I've managed to persuade College that its nurse Glynis should undergo training as a counsellor – a long process for her, but one she's keen to go through. It's a breakthrough for the pastoral system here. We've been struggling with a number of problem cases among the students and we don't have enough Fellows who are able or willing to help out with giving advice. Having a trained counsellor on site will help the whole community to feel supported and to function better.

Diary of a Bipolar Explorer

March 2005: Weightwatchers

The spring weather is here; our *magnolia stellata* is in full bloom, its white stars profuse. The bulbs are up among the grass in the Library garden in College.

There's nothing so fulfilling as watching my weight drop away; nothing so satisfying as the public weigh-in, the plaudits, the little rewards. I love my trips to Weightwatchers, the camaraderie with women who are doing the same. I enjoy waiting in the queue to be weighed – the chat, the support, the laughter. This is the fourth time in my life that I've been able to transform my body. It's like a sculpture on which I'm working steadily. I see it taking a new shape almost as if it's separate from me. The goal of five stones weight-loss is eventually achieved but this isn't the only gratification; there's also an addiction in the daily weighing at home, the graphs, the self-congratulations. The gym too is a form of addiction. I'm getting so good at keeping fit that it takes over many hours in the week and is becoming the main focus of my thoughts. I get a high from this. After three years without alcohol I no longer miss that kind of elation. The exercise is far superior – my creativity goes into the image of my body.

Chapter Two: The Aftermath

April 2005: Joy

The apple trees are in blossom; the days are lengthening; summer is already in the air. There's a phrase, "to be beside oneself with joy" which I understand. It's as if I'm two people, one experiencing it and one watching myself doing so. "Pleasure" isn't a big enough word for the exhilaration of knowing that I can walk tall. Elation is much nearer the mark. It feels almost dangerous that I'm so excited, doing without sleep yet feeling energised. I bound up the stairs; all spaces are clearings. I share in the spring; it becomes a part of me.

Spring 2005: Overwork

My edition of Edward Thomas's *Oxford* is published by Signal Books – the result of many months of research. I'm drawn to Thomas partly because of my recent interest in literature of the First World War, partly because I identify with him as a depressive prose-writer who turned latterly to poetry. Working on his prose I realise that a big multi-volume edition of his prose works is much needed; this must happen next. I'm frenetically busy co-organising a conference on Thomas which brings academics and poets together.

Diary of a Bipolar Explorer

As always with community projects involving poetry there's a heady excitement in the air. I've lost sight of what a sensible workload is and my energy levels seem to be soaring. Is this what is meant by "hypomania"? If so, I like it! Should I be getting help from someone for this dangerous feeling which is a bit like being on a coffee high?

June 2005: Shopping

I feel uneasy. I should be getting help, but I keep putting it off. To have transformed my shape is one thing; to display it another. I go shopping every day, heading out at lunchtime to search for something new, something that will suit me and show off my transformed self. The high is short-lived; the money feels thrown away almost as soon as it's spent. I'm running up debts. I can easily spend £500 in a single day. I'm addicted to this new person I've created. I look at myself in the mirror and scarcely know the image as myself. I've become a kind of mannequin. Why are there so many clothes in my wardrobe that I'll never wear? Some of them still have their price labels on. I can't count how much all this has cost me. Martin bails me out, watching anxiously.

Chapter Two: The Aftermath

July 2005: Publication

They say that having a book published is like giving birth; I haven't found it to be so joyous until now, though I've known previous publications to be long drawn out and painful like a birth. Having *Ginnel* appear in print is perhaps the proudest moment of my life – much more so than becoming a Professor. I wish dad and Sally could be here to share my pleasure. But of course I could never have become a poet without their deaths. It was the pain of Sally's dying that got me started writing poetry for the first time and it was in the aftermath of dad's death that I wrote *Ginnel*. How strange to find myself feeling a kind of gratitude for loss.

The trip to Leeds to give a public reading at my book launch fills me with fear. I'm getting no better with experience at travelling or publicly performing. And yet when I do stand up to read I feel more confident about my poems than I do in lectures, as if the whole of me is present. Something new is happening; I feel more integrated than I've felt for a long while.

Diary of a Bipolar Explorer

October 2005: Memories

The seasons have their own rhythms and so too does the family calendar, studded with the anniversaries of deaths. Always, in the months between October and December, my mind is with the memory of Sally's last months alive. I can recall the unfolding illness in graphic detail. As Christmas nears each day holds the sharp imprint of the end of 1999, as if I'm living in double time. Grieving is a long-drawn out process and I realise there are many years of remembering still to come. My father died in October, so two family deaths go on being intertwined in my memories. It's hard to concentrate on other things while processing these. I inhabit the past very intensively.

February 2006: Academic pressures

Call for papers. Academic Committee agenda. Examiners' meeting. Call for papers. College Committee agenda. Call for papers. Draft papers for FHS English. Faculty Meeting agenda. Call for papers. Governing Body agenda. Call for papers. Timetable for Collections... The emails are incessant, the pressure to publish intense. Anyone who thinks that Oxford academics have an easy life should think again.

Chapter Two: The Aftermath

The days of quiet individual research in libraries are long over. Tutorial Fellows have two employers – the University and College – competing for their time and attention. Research productivity jostles with the demands of teaching and administration; pastoral duties can sometimes be neglected in the rush to get things done; social obligations in College and University add extra pressures. Colleagues rush around, heads to the ground – no time to stop and chat, no time to notice that that the days are already getting longer, that the snowdrops are in bloom, that daffodils are pushing their heads up around the trees. Lunchtime conversation is perfunctory. Marking must be taken home and done in the evenings and weekends. There's no space for writing the articles and books that are expected and young academics take on teaching burdens that older academics are impatient with carrying. I'm a Professor now but with no change in duties and no secretarial help. We're short-staffed in my subject, with a large number of students – and tutorials (though enjoyable as always) are draining. I bury myself in routine work, trying to fulfil all my contractual obligations. I decline invitations to give papers at conferences. Enough is enough.

June 2006: Another death

I feel numbed by the death of my former husband Jonathan. We remained friends after our divorce, though we lost touch latterly. I knew it was coming but I was excluded by family circumstances from seeing him before he died very suddenly leaving his grief-stricken wife with two small children and a baby. I've heard from others about the funeral in Dorset, in the village where we used to have a cottage. I remember the columbine and buddleia-filled garden, our walks from the cottage to the cliff for views of the sea. One day I'll make a pilgrimage to his grave to take in the fact of his dying. How strange to go over and over a shared life that's doubly finished – by divorce and by death. His wife has left some things of his in my pigeonhole, including a first edition of Wordsworth's *Poems, 1815*, with a pencilled inscription for me on the inside front cover. It's very touching to have a lasting memento. It will be years before I can process what this death means. I feel very still.

September 2006: A milestone

I'm back from a weekend in Venice with Martin and Emma – we went for a family holiday, to celebrate my fiftieth birthday. It couldn't have been lovelier; even the pelting rain was romantic in this city of water and moving reflections. We were enchanted by the gondolas, the flaking dilapidated buildings sinking into the lagoon. We loved the Museum of Modern Art, the paintings in dark churches, the little back streets – and the student quarter, where we found some amazing book-shops and bought some intricately crafted sweets made of multi-coloured glass. The Piazza was flooded while we were there, but nothing put us off our delight in this ancient city. We went round the Doges' Palace and admired the portraits of long sinister faces. The only sadness on my birthday (when we ate a delicious lunch of fresh fish outside in a thankfully sunlit square) was the knowledge that Sally hadn't reached fifty. I'm not able to talk with her on the phone about all the things we saw, all the fun we had walking about the streets and taking rides on gondolas. She would have loved to hear.

October 2006: The anxiety of reception

In addition to undergraduate tuition, research and graduate supervision, I give two eight-week courses of lectures in the University each year. Here I am at the age of fifty, an experienced academic with twenty-five years of teaching behind me, yet I'm still sleepless the night before I stand up before an audience to speak. Nor does the problem end there, because I go over and over each lecture in my head once it's over, finding fault with every performance. I've always found lecturing a challenge but the difficulties have become extreme since Sally died. (I used to talk to her about lecturing; like my dad she was a great communicator and seemed entirely at ease when standing up and talking. She always told me to relax and do without notes – fat chance of that when you're bipolar, but it was good advice. No-one wants to listen to a lecturer who can't *ad lib*.)

Back in 2000, I published a book about Romantic writers and their defensive reactions to the rise of a mass reading-public and professional criticism. In tracking what I called their "anxiety of reception" was I projecting onto these writers my own pathology? Certainly it's the number and unfamiliarity of people in a University audience that frightens me. I feel alienated by their staring eyes, their fingers tapping my words into their laptops. There's something anonymous and perfunctory in our interaction. By contrast, in College classes and tutorials with my own students I feel no anxiety. Teaching just two students at a time I can have a real conversation with them.

CHAPTER TWO: THE AFTERMATH

I've written this poem to celebrate the bond that forms with my students through teaching. Tutorials are the centre of my working day, and my main source of professional fulfilment:

The Tutorial

When all else fails, when
other joys are stifled or blocked,
there's this. There is always this.

Not a road and a railway
but a passage and a bridge;
not the lines of travel, but the junction.

Not coordinates and a map
but a path and a missing turn;
not arrival, but direction.

Not a whetstone and a knife
but a basket and its weave;
not combat, but connection.

Not luck and the solitary search
but a step and a link,
not the catch, but the cognition.

Not an argument and its conclusion
but a craft and its pattern,
not invention but elucidation.

Not a quiz and its solution
but a query, a suggestion;
not repartee but conversation.

Not a method and a programme
but a habit and a way of life;
not duty, but vocation.

Not pilgrims and a guide
but companions on a road;
not instruction but communication.

Not closure, but perfect timing:
a voice on the stair, a knock on the door –
something nearing completion.

February 2007: College life

A louring sky over ivory towers; it's bitterly cold as I cycle over Magdalen Bridge at rush hour. Medieval institutions press in all around; I feel benighted. Going through the gate into College in the morning is like entering a cave full of people casting shadows from a light whose source can't be located. The shadows flit and elongate; it's hard to tell where substance thins into shadow.

Oxford colleges are like dysfunctional families. The community is small, with a *paterfamilias* and sibling rivalries; there's infighting and squabbling. Every member of a college brings to the workplace their own family history and projects onto their colleagues and friends the problems they experienced as a child. Every conversation, every action, is distorted by the presence of emotional activity that lies well beyond communal control. We the Fellows are interpreters, reading each other's family histories behind the actions that we take and the ways that we perform. We each have problems with hearing what the other says. Sometimes we watch each other speak as if we're lip-reading.

June 2007: Stress

It's like a hammer banging again and again inside my head, or a trapped bird inside my chest, beating its angry wings. When it's there for any length of time it paralyses. Experiencing it repeatedly wears the mind down. There's too much of it at work. I can't get a grip on it; it's hard to stand back from, hard to think or write about clearly. This is no way to live; I don't even have time to read a newspaper.

Diary of a Bipolar Explorer

August 2007: China

We've been away from home for three weeks on a nature tour in China which took us from Heathrow to Beijing then on to Chengdu and Kunming, ending with a couple of days in Hong Kong. There was very little nature in sight until we reached the beautiful countryside at Lijiang and visited Tiger Leaping Gorge, two highlights of the tour. We moved with the guides from hotel to hotel, our every action closely supervised and with little time to wander off on our own. Emma was enchanted with the pandas at Wolong, I with the Great Wall, where we got the exercise and the vistas of country that I was craving. Martin was curious, fascinated by and enjoying everything. The heat was overpowering and in Beijing we were unable to see the sun for thick fog. Everywhere we went we were astonished by the number of people hurrying about the streets in crowds. Being away from home for so long, struggling to understand Chinese culture, was immensely challenging. I was oppressed by reading Jung Chang's great family saga, *Wild Swans: Three Daughters of China* and by looking all around me at the poverty in which people are living. On every coach journey my mind was divided between the history of Communism I found in the book and the depredations of industrialisation that I could see from the coach window. The absence of familiar landmarks and familiar language disoriented me. I succumbed to culture shock and found myself shaking and crying at the airport between two legs of our trip.

I became aware of the full extent of my depression after a coach journey out into the mountains to see the nature reserve at Jiuzhaigou. Here I was convinced that the whole area was completely devoid of any wildlife; pollution had so destroyed China that all that remained was the landscape itself. Was the whole place a film-set, a simulacrum for tourists? There were many dead trees, fallen into the lake or strewn around it; no birds in the branches of the woods; and only a few wild flowers to suggest a thriving habitat. A single butterfly landed within my viewfinder. I snapped it eagerly.

On returning to Oxford we've learnt that our former colleague, the philosopher Susan Hurley, has died. Susan was a true friend and my age – we even shared a birthday. I walk behind the library, where I used to go with her and find the garden dug up, ready to be re-designed. "Long live the weeds and the wilderness yet": Gerard Manley Hopkins' poem echoes in my mind as I walk back through the graveyard sadly.

Diary of a Bipolar Explorer

October 2007: Sick leave

Oh God, not the black dog *again*. Every day, all day. There's a corner of the bed – deep in under the duvet, near to the hot-water bottle – which is the only place to be as Michaelmas Term looms and the autumn days shorten. How I long to stay in there, with no call on my time and attention. Motherhood is demanding too much of me and I feel I'm failing on every front. My marriage is under strain. The summer has given me no break from myself and the trip to China has opened up a gulf in my feelings which I find hard to fathom. Returning to Oxford to learn of Susan's death was shocking; the more I think about it, the more symbolic resonance attaches to the ploughed-up land at the back of the graveyard. I've been restless and miserable, unable to concentrate on my work. Now I'm plummeting very rapidly into clinical depression.

I've been signed off sick for three months. My doctor has put me on medication and referred me to the Warneford for a consultation. It's years since I've been there. I dread it.

February 2008: The Consultant

He's so very urbane. And a magician! He can scroll through the case history with a single flick of his finger.

CHAPTER TWO: THE AFTERMATH

Simultaneously (and in real time) he can watch it flow past on his monitor while shuffling the notes on his big shiny desk to home in on the salient features... And he can do all this in the patient's presence while smiling, joking, as if it the whole thing were some midsummer lark!

Meanwhile – quietly, with no fuss – he checks out the true state of affairs with one or two unexpected questions out of the blue. And out of the blue the larks are ascending. The patient can watch them from this very room by focusing on a small patch of window. They fly high, way above this hospital and on, over the road, over the playground, the park, the Sheldonian, the colleges, the

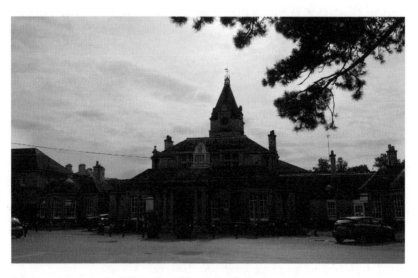

Main entrance to the Warneford Hospital, Oxford

university, the multi-storey car park, the castle, the prison, the railway-station, the canal, the allotments, the pub, the quiet lanes to Binsey…

Are they there still? Were they ever there? The Consultant has stopped talking now. The appointment is over. Don't expect a record of what took place. It's strictly confidential.

June 2008: The questionnaires

They send me the same questionnaires every Monday. The data from both of them go into a double graph, which helps to build a picture of recurring patterns in my mood disorder. This is how I answered the multiple choice questions this week on the first of the questionnaires:

Depression

I take more than 60 minutes to fall asleep, more than half the time

I awaken more than once a night and stay awake for 20 minutes or more, more than half the time

I awaken at least one hour before I need to, and can't go back to sleep

I feel sad more than half the time

Chapter Two: The Aftermath

There is no change in my usual appetite
I have not had a change in my weight
Most of the time I struggle to focus my attention or to
make decisions
I largely believe that I cause problems for others
I do not think of suicide or death

*

Years ago they asked whether I'd describe it as a
mood or a feeling.
It's both.
They asked what it feels like.
In the mornings a wall; in the afternoons a tunnel; in
the evenings a sticky envelope.
They asked if it ever gets better.
It's always there. The sticky envelope is better than the wall.
They asked if there's anything that might help it,
anything from outside.
There isn't an outside.
They asked what I thought it was.
I looked at the wall.
I asked what they thought it was.

Diary of a Bipolar Explorer

Mania

This is the second questionnaire they send me every Monday. It's briefer. The data go into the same graph but in a different colour. I can't describe its shape. This is how I filled it in this week:

I often feel happier or more cheerful than usual
I often feel more self-confident than usual
I often need less sleep than usual
I frequently talk more than is usual
I have frequently been more active than usual

A long time ago they asked whether I'd describe it as a mood or a feeling.
It's both.
They asked what it's like.
Joy, hope, love, breath, communication, a drench of sunshine, sitting under the apple tree, high wind on the moors, a long open vista, energy that will never end; poetry in song, rhythm in poetry. Happiness that pierces and dissolves; the sense that everything is mysteriously connected.

They asked does anything make it better.

It's already the best there is.

They asked why I want it to go on.

Who wouldn't?

They asked if anything helps it, anything from outside.

There isn't an outside.

They asked what I thought it was.

You tell me.

They said we're going to send you two questionnaires to fill in each week.

Why two? I'm one person.

July 2008: The double graph

At the consultation – just one consultation, you understand, because I'm one person – we look at the double graph. There's no pattern to the depression line, which is a long low trail with a few peaks like whisked egg, some of them exactly coinciding with peaks in the mania line but mostly doing their own thing. The mania line has jumped right away from the other one a month earlier, done a bit of a dance, and is still soaring.

DIARY OF A BIPOLAR EXPLORER

Although it's curiously de-humanising to see one's moods mapped out in these wavering lines, I try to identify myself as two halves of one person when I look at the double graph and think of them both as equally intriguing. *I go back a long way; I'm split in two – but they're both myself.*

My consultant is usually interested, as he is on this occasion, only in the mania line – and in stopping any hypomanic peaks from worsening. By contrast, I'm invariably committed, against my own best interests, to keeping those peaks going for as long as I can. What is the point of the consultation? For him to wear down my stubborn resistance? For me to triumph secretly over his professional firmness?

"Why resist the medication?" he asks.

I don't want this phase to end. I'm getting stuff done. It happens so rarely. Most of all I love the night-watch, when everything comes into focus, in bed or at my desk; thoughts reaching into silence.

He explains the importance of sleep, the danger of psychosis. While he's talking I'm lost in thought, drafting a letter of protest to the highest authorities about the dehumanising reductiveness of the double graph. Will it ever be sent?

Dear Highest Authorities,

I object to undergoing a process of surveillance which I feel to be reductive. As you can see from my writing (which I attach) I have strong reservations about filling in Multiple Choice Questionnaires. I resent being kept under observation. I dislike being split in two by psychiatrists and reduced to two lines on a graph. If I really must be watched by myself and the doctors all the time, I would prefer a more integrative questionnaire, especially as the pattern of my illness involves episodes of "mixed" mood at both extremes. Sometimes it's hard to fill in these questionnaires, as the moods alter so rapidly – even within a single day. Although there may be excellent research reasons for collecting information in this way, they don't help me, the patient. I've been filling in these questionnaires for a while – the graph is already so long...where and what am I in it?

Yours sincerely,
LN

The consultation's over. He can see my mind is on something else, something more important. He switches off the monitor. We can no longer see the double graph. "Keep filling in the weekly questionnaires," he encourages

71

briskly as I collect the two strands of myself together to leave – "and here's the prescription. I'll see you again in a few months' time."

On the way out I meet a colleague in the waiting room – he's there to see the same consultant. The knowledge of our common bipolar condition, secretly shared in a professional environment, makes the afternoon worthwhile. Fellow-feeling even goes some way towards offsetting annoyance with myself for not sending off the letter. I imagine my colleague sitting in the seat I've just sat in and a vision comes to me of the university's entire academic staff staring at themselves reduced to double graphs on multiple monitors. It's a vision so pleasing in its absurdity that I know I'll be revisiting it in the early hours of the morning. I walk home humming Pete Seeger's "Little Boxes".

Chapter Three:
Crisis

It isn't hard work that makes the years so grim but grief and the illness worsening and nowhere to hide from duties of every kind and no energy to play. This is no way to bring up a child. It isn't the workplace that makes me sleepless but my condition worsening and nowhere to bring up a child away from duties of every kind and no energy to play. This is no way to be. It isn't College that drains me of all vitality but the conditions under which I'm living: myself partly my own employer, my husband at the same college as me and nowhere to hide from my child and no energy to work or play. This is no way for a marriage to be. It isn't disloyalty that makes me resent my employers, but the conditions under which I've been working and nowhere to hide from duties of every kind and no-one to blame but me. It isn't grievance that makes the years so dark but grief and my illness worsening and nowhere to hide from myself, my own employer. This is no way to bring up a child. This is no way to be.

Diary of a Bipolar Explorer

And so it goes on until I snap one day, outing my condition at work as no way to be: something, I explain, *has never been acknowledged.* I rail against my employer, who is partly me. It isn't College that makes me manic but the illness worsening and nowhere to conceal my duties and no way I can bring up a child, or play. It isn't duty that makes these years so grim but depression and a grievance worsening and nowhere to hide from work of every kind. This is no way for a family to be. It isn't duty of any kind, or conditions at work, or lack of energy to play that makes it no way to be, but the grievance of death and mania and the illness worsening…till the child turns and rails at me.

December 2008: The stolen dossier

I've been robbed, coming along Old Road. The experience was so shocking that I'm still trembling. The police took an immensely long time to turn up. I doubt if they'll ever retrieve my bag which contains, in a single dossier, all the materials relating to my illness and difficulties in College… I don't care about the £300 in cash which I had in my purse for Christmas shopping, or the bag itself, which will be covered by insurance. All I care about is my confidential dossier. I feel devastated. When the words come, they are in verse. Only through rhyme and rhythm can I convey the shock:

A car slowed down, a sudden hand reached out,
grabbing my bag and driving swiftly on.
It was broad daylight. I began to shout,
but no one heard; she was already gone.

Grabbing my bag and driving swiftly on,
she turned to clock me with triumphant eyes.
But no one saw; she was already gone,
gloating no doubt over her stolen prize.

She turned to clock me with triumphant eyes;
I'll not forget the way they pierced me through.
Gloating no doubt over her stolen prize
she left me stunned, unsure of what to do.

I'll not forget the way they pierced me through,
those eyes that now could pore over my life.
She left me stunned, unsure of what to do;
exposed to view, as if skinned by a knife.

Those eyes that now could pore over my life
would know by now my dossier's secret shame −

exposed to view, as if skinned by a knife;
would know my grievance, and my need to blame.

She'd know by now my dossier's secret shame,
my mental illness and my lasting grief.
She'd know my grievance and my need to blame.
She left me broken, stripped – a skeleton leaf.

My mental illness and my lasting grief,
could they be read now, by more pairs of eyes?
She left me broken, stripped – a skeleton leaf;
raw, and a prey to others' prying lies.

Would they be read now, by more pairs of eyes?
It was broad daylight. I began to shout,
raw, and a prey to others' prying lies.
a car slowed down, a sudden hand reached out.

December 2008: Rumour

I'm obsessed with the fear that my dossier may have been picked up by someone who will spread the confidential documents or sell my story to a newspaper, bringing disgrace to me, my family and College. I keep trying to reassure myself that all the thief wanted was my purse but I can't help feeling intensely exposed. Again I turn to poetry for relief and self-expression. The pantoum, with its strange circling refrains, is a vehicle for obsessional thoughts:

Where has it gone, my own voice speaking?
What are these words now travelling fast,
what is this thing I hear repeating,
calling and beating like gulls in the mist?

What are these words now travelling fast,
filling the air with strange dark sounds,
calling and beating like gulls in the mist,
spreading the news of mutual wounds?

Filling the air with strange dark sounds
the message (no longer a muffled murmur)
releasing the news of mutual wounds
is now a rumble of garbled rumour.

The message (no longer a muffled murmur —
reaching beyond me, its echoes vast)
is now the rumble of garbled rumour
and mangled meanings, their origin lost.

Reaching beyond me (its echoes vast
now I am prey to others' dark humour

and mangled meanings, their origin lost)
stigma is forming a sturdy tumour.

Now I am prey to others' dark humour,
what is this thing I hear repeating?
Stigma is forming a sturdy tumour.
Where has it gone, my own voice speaking?

January 2009: Worsening

Under the duvet is the only place to be. I've felt worse over Christmas. It's impossible to concentrate, impossible to work. I can't move around in College without thinking about how my illness affects the way I relate to others. How many people know what my condition is? How does my illness change my role? What are the limits of empathy among those who have to work with me? How many others are there with disabilities who feel the same sense of stigma that I am feeling – or worse?

Stigma

Closing round an open wound
it grips, and takes a stubborn hold.
It reaches in, behind, around
and spreads like mildew, moss, or mould.

It grips, and takes a stubborn hold
on all that has been done or said.
It spreads like mildew, moss or mould
And fills a life with silent dread.

In all that has been done or said
it finds new sustenance, and so
it fills a life with silent dread,
growing as far as it can grow.

It finds new sustenance and so
it thickens, like a wall of pain
growing as far as it can grow
to spread its toxins like a stain.

It thickens like a wall of pain.
It reaches in, behind, around
to spread its toxins like a stain,
Closing round an open wound.

March 2009: Looking for help

I have some good friends who are sympathetic, helping me to feel less isolated. (Nicky, where would I be without your affection and support?) But in general, why is it so difficult to communicate with colleagues about mental health? Is there a double standard? Would they listen more attentively if the illness was physical? I'm involved now in a complicated conversation with College about how best to deal with my disability. I feel angry and upset that this has never been fully acknowledged. I disclosed my condition when first diagnosed, but there was no discussion at the time about the implications. Has this made my condition worse? I'm obsessed with the idea that a letter was sent from St James's Hospital to tell the College authorities about my psychotic breakdown. Again the obsession finds an outlet in poetry:

The missing letter

Somehow, somewhere, something has been lost.
I thrash about, not knowing who to blame.
My past life's mine no more, a frantic ghost.

Where is that letter when it's needed most?
I'm sure they wrote it, and I think it came.
Somehow, somewhere, something has been lost.

I rail against mischance − the useless post −
all normal explanations seeming lame.
My past life's mine no more, a frantic ghost.

The proof of what I did's not much to boast;
I'd like it here in writing all the same
that something then was broken down, and lost.

Who is there left that I can really trust?
"Duty of Care" is just an empty name.
My past life's mine no more – a frantic ghost,

a parasite that's eaten by its host,
a piece of trash that others can defame.
Somehow, somewhere, something has been lost.

I cannot calculate the final cost
of all that will be wagered in this game.
My past life's mine no more, a frantic ghost;

and what is left is buried in the dust,
with no one but myself to feel the shame.
Somehow, somewhere, something has been lost -
my past life's mine no more, a frantic ghost.

March 2009 Asylum Welcome

Help has come in the form of a wider perspective. I'm involved in an exciting project organised by Brookes University in association with Oxford's Asylum Welcome.

DIARY OF A BIPOLAR EXPLORER

It's a community project bringing poets together with asylum-seekers to create a book. I'm working with an Eritrean woman and her daughter on a pair of poems which will be published alongside each other. Hers is an expression of pride in her daughter's amazing skills as a champion ice-skater; mine is prompted by losing my passport and remembering Uganda, where I was born. My lost passport has triggered a crisis of identity (possibly connected with the theft of my confidential dossier) and my memories come back thick and fast. I'm newly troubled by recollections of the Amin regime, but getting to know Eden and Hegen is one of the best things in my recent life. Crafting my poem and helping to improve the English in Eden's raises my spirits and makes me feel part of a wider world. I'm learning a great deal about the suffering of refugees.

May-June 2009: Madness

There's a strange clarity to all my thoughts, as if I'm hallucinating. I feel that I'm beginning to lose my mind. Terror of insanity grips me. I've become obsessed with chronology and yet scarcely know which day of the week it is. My current appointments and teaching duties flicker past me as if in a film or dream. I live in the past, mapping out a narrative of my illness. I feel that my underlying condition has been exacerbated by stress and understaffing. College should understand my difficulties, so that reasonable adjustments can be made and future cases of disability handled more coherently. Persuading my colleagues of this involves a painstaking resuscitation of past episodes of illness mapped onto a timeline of the university's calendar over the last seven years. Drawing on clinical records to back up my arguments I ask doctors to corroborate my accounts. I email colleagues reminding them of their duty of care. I visit Occupational Health. I even go to the local University and Colleges Union rep. for legal and practical advice. I'm reassured by the kindness of the professionals I encounter as I get to understand my own mental health issues in a wider context. My activities are focused on a mission which is personally motivated but which I see as having benefits for the community at large. I don't want anyone in future with a disability to go through such difficulties.

I'm hypomanic and driven but also depressed and angry: it would be impossible to capture the mixture of moods in a single phrase. I suppose I'm looking for someone or something in the system to blame. My grievance is inseparable from grief; I memorialise the self that has been suppressed for seven years, struggling behind a mask of professional success. My obsession becomes so extreme that what goes on in the garden is forgotten: I scarcely notice the summer. This is the nearest I've ever been to feeling suicidal. And yet I go through the motions of living. I talk with Emma about school, I go to the gym, play squash with a friend. I take out my frustration on the ball with strong swipes of the racket. (Nicky, our squash-games and cups of coffee are a lifeline. Without your sanity I would be lost.)

I've been seeing a counsellor, who's cool and brisk. I like the dispassionate way in which she reminds me that others go through similar difficulties; that there are structures in place which will lend support. For the first time I've had professional help in revisiting the psychotic episode in Leeds. She has enabled me to see that this was a small-scale domestic matter, badly handled by us as a family. In the same way, perhaps I'm enlarging a personal grudge against College into an injustice? Wasn't it my own obligation to take care of my mental health? How can College be held responsible for what is a personal crisis? Why am I so obsessed with a lost document which paid attention to my psychotic episode if it's not that, at some level, I feel guilty about having neglected myself? My illness is shrunk to its real size by my counsellor's sensible down-to-earth questions. Talking with her of my preoccupation with chronology and timelines we've looked together at the double graphs charting my mood swings and recognised a monthly pattern in them. Is there something in my condition that is worsened by the menopause? Am I subject to the ghostly vestiges of a monthly cycle? I've been speculating and have found evidence in some books that Bipolar Disorder can be exacerbated by this biological transition.

The best help I find for myself is in writing. When I go to my computer to write a letter of complaint I train myself to switch into my collection of poems, *Earth's Almanac*, where I'm telling the story of Sally's death through seasonal change. Here I use nature's timeline, the calendar, to ground my life. I find myself split between the pastoral solace I find in the seasons and the absurd brokenness of my illness narrative. How come I'm writing about the natural world so attentively while at the same time oblivious to what is going on in our garden? Which summer is it that I'm writing about in my poems? Where am I on this double graph of illness mapped out month by month? How many timelines am I constructing?

85

Diary of a Bipolar Explorer

Every attempt to understand what's happening to me goes back remorselessly to two key events: my sister's and my father's deaths. The second I can accept; the first I'll never get over. My poetry becomes intensely elegiac, all the more so because I'm using it to surmount the difficulties I have with understanding the passage of time. Yet again a period of creativity – writing every day and long into the night – is both the product of insanity and my way of remaining sane.

June 2009: Damaged relationships

It's hot. I spend too many hours at my desk in College or at home, emailing about my medical condition and its implications. One of the worst aspects of this illness is the havoc it wreaks on relationships. I've found nothing in any of the books on bipolarity that helps. I've lost two important friendships at work; there's no consolation apart from other friendships that deepen – and Martin's love, which remains constant through thick and thin. There have been times when our marriage has been under strain because of the onset of episodes. This has been the worst stretch of instability I've experienced since 2002. Matters are made worse, not better, by the fact that we work in the same place and never escape our duties to College. Sometimes I honestly don't know how he copes.

CHAPTER THREE: CRISIS

June 2009: The night editor – a dream

I've become fearful of surveillance and dread the loss of my own identity as I try to make sense of what is happening to me. My nights are mostly sleepless. Last night I had a short spell of fitful sleep in which I had this dream about an authority figure tampering with my documents:

> *There he was in the low light, with the shadow from the bookcase on the carpet slightly swaying. He sat at my desk with his back to me. And as I paused in the doorway I knew that he had come to read my words in secrecy. But as I stood watching him at my desk, leaning over my keyboard with my documents on screen, I saw that he was mostly typing.*
>
> *There he was and as I came further in he stopped his quiet tapping to turn slowly in my chair so I could see his face. He smiled and by his smile I knew him. Then he turned away and continued tapping. The sound was louder now, less secretive. I stood for a long while watching him – my words disappearing from the screen; his hands with slender fingers, typing.*
>
> *There he was and I stood sickened. There he was and I knew who he was and I watched his words filling up the spaces where mine had been and I knew what he was changing. And as I woke, I knew this was no dream.*

Diary of a Bipolar Explorer

July 2009: The meeting

I can't go on living at this pitch of anxiety. I've made representations and had an initial meeting with a few senior colleagues. Now my case – I won't call it a formal complaint, it isn't that – is coming up for consideration at Governing Body. I've given advance notice that I may not be able to attend the meeting. I feel unbalanced and fear that stress may get the better of me. But still I prepare myself as best as I can, intending to go.

My heart pounds and my mouth is dry as I face a room full of colleagues. I keep my words to a minimum and focus on points of general principle. I point out that there are sometimes conflicts of interest that arise from being a Fellow and therefore a member of Governing Body. I discuss how difficult it is to be one's own employer and to find the right mechanisms to monitor and make allowance for disability. I explain that I've had a grievance with College – which includes myself, my own employer – about how my disability has been handled. There has been a long correspondence about this; several people in the room know about it already. There are questions. The meeting is finished quickly. The Fellows have listened and given me what I asked for. They've behaved well. The struggle is over. I feel reassured that in future the proper measures will be in place. Something good will come out of all this.

It felt throughout as if a strong white light was shining directly at me while I talked. I felt raw and exposed. As my mouth opened and shut I could hear cogent sentences coming out; but I was separate from this – I was back in St James's Hospital, being questioned about my identity. Walking away from the meeting, I'm in two places at once and strangely disconnected from my body.

August 2009: The Eye

It creeps up on me gradually. There isn't just one, looking particularly malicious in the full light of day. They're everywhere in College, glaring or squinting at me. "We installed them for Security Reasons," the Bursar explains. I try to forget.

For a while I put it down to coincidence. Then I observe that if I've had a ropey day at work there's invariably an email the next day advertising *hidden* cameras – not the visible security ones but high-tech spy cameras for secret surveillance purposes. I often break into a cold sweat as I sort through my inbox. I take to checking the light-fittings in my office for suspicious objects. I'm unable to sleep for three nights after watching *The Sixth Sense*. It isn't the ghost that's frightening but the revelation of a hidden camera observing the bedroom where the child has been gradually, secretly, poisoned by her mother.

One day, working at home, I notice there's a small fleck at the centre of my computer screen. It looks round – more and more round as the day wears on. It's white against blue with a dark centre like a tiny pupil. I could swear it clocks me when I leave my desk; I could swear it follows my movements to and fro all morning from document to document, in and out of emails. I'm trying to concentrate on writing a confidential letter relating to my recent ill health. Every word I write is being watched by the fleck, so I get nothing done.

By lunchtime I've convinced myself it's a spy camera, installed by the College to observe me at home. But perhaps there's a reasonable explanation; perhaps it's some kind of virus, or bug? I ring the Computing Services:

Is it possible there's a bug in my computer?

What does it look like, and what does it do?

It's like a small eye, at the centre of the screen. It seems to move; it seems to watch me.

How small, and have you tried cleaning the monitor?

Smaller than a lentil; and the monitor is clean.

Bring it in, we'll take a look and try to reassure you.

90

Chapter Three: Crisis

Try to reassure me. Without delay I get into the car. In town I park and forget to feed the meter. I walk into the entrance of Computer Services. I walk fast because by this stage I've become convinced that someone's following me; he will hang around outside till I re-emerge. I explain about the fleck to a nice man, keeping my voice as matter of fact as possible; it wouldn't do to convey too much panic. He checks my laptop, updates my Sophos protection, and smiles as though my fear is an average everyday occurrence; as though it's to be expected that employees will assume they are being observed at home by a spy camera. I'm sweating by the time I leave to find the car. There's someone following me for sure. I can't find the car, I can't remember where I parked it. Eventually it turns up with a parking-fine attached to the screen. I pull away sharply.

What possesses me to drop into College? I don't know. I convince myself I need to retrieve a confidential document relating to my health from the computer in my room. I've shaken off whoever was following me, but when I arrive in my room it's clear someone has been in there searching for something. For a week or so I've been wondering about the light-fittings, whether they might allow concealment of spy cameras. This evening I re-check them, climbing on a chair to unscrew each bulb and replace it with a new one. By now the sweating is a problem and my heart is pounding. It isn't like the fear you feel at night, having convinced yourself the noise you heard was a burglar. It's a much more pervasive fear that the whole room is under surveillance and bugged.

There's only one place where I feel I'm unobserved – in the adjoining loo. There I can close the door and read the document as soon as I've found it and printed it out. Every one of my actions is visible to my observers while in the main room, but in the loo-room I'm safe. I preserve a dignified bearing, moving in an unhurried fashion between the rooms. When I'm sure the document is the one I need I leave my room, locking it carefully, and go down to talk to the porters:

Someone has been in my room, I'd like to get the locks changed.

What makes you think that?

Things have been moved.

Could that be your scout? (A scout is the Oxford name for cleaner.)

She doesn't move my stuff.

When do you think this happened?

Last night for sure.

We can double check.

How?

We can watch everything that happened last night in the front quad on this screen. We can play it back on film, you can watch it with us. We have a security camera trained on the entrance to your staircase.

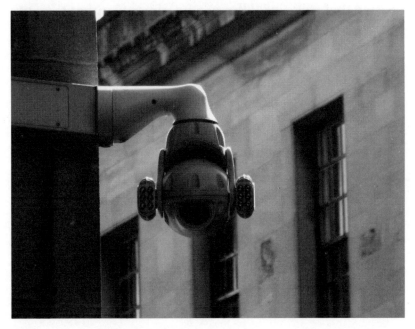

Security camera, Library Garden St Edmund Hall (photo by Peter J. King)

August 2009: A strange summer

The after-effects of that Governing Body meeting are becoming apparent. I'm laid open by the exposure and feel watched by the whole community at work. Fortunately this is vacation time so there are few people around, but I do have to drop into College sometimes and always there's the sense of surveillance.

Yesterday, visited in College by my nephew Mike, I insisted that we have coffee in a nearby café rather than my room because of the hidden cameras. He looked at me as if I was mad (as I am) but he fell in with my paranoia, and we were able to talk freely in the café. I've even insisted that Martin double-checks the light-fittings for me. In all this I'm aware of how ludicrous and far-fetched my anxieties must seem to someone who's outside my consciousness. Fear of insanity is worse than being insane.

September 2009: The Torch Man

I'm back from a month in Cornwall. Only now am I able to process what went on and to turn it into a kind of story. By doing this I make it a little less terrifying. Here's what happened.

The lane dropped steeply, turning in a hairpin bend round the house. It was perfect: a converted barn hidden in a valley with a door opening onto woods. A secluded path ran beside a stream through dense woodland to the sea. I'd have a month of isolation – days writing and walking, nights listening to the owls.

Chapter Three: Crisis

There were two or three houses just along from the one I'd rented – but they were all holiday homes and at this stage empty. I wasn't use to being on my own and from the very first day felt apprehensive. So tense had I been in the preceding month that my counsellor had suggested I call her regularly on the phone while in Cornwall to keep her in touch with my state of mind. There was no land-line. The signal for my mobile was almost non-existent. I would be able to ride my bike into the village and call her and my family from there; but down in this dark valley I truly was alone.

There were no curtains on the skylights in the bedroom. I worked out immediately that if you stood on the lane rising behind the house you could look in at me sleeping. There wasn't a soul in sight all day long in this lone stretch of countryside and yet I was haunted by fear of a peeping Tom. I searched hurriedly for anything that might make the bedroom a little more private, but gave up, defeated; the barn was kitted out in Spartan fashion and the owners were clearly used to clients who liked to live as much in the wild as they could.

If Martin had been with me we would doubtless have looked forward to lying in bed gazing up at the night sky. We would have kept the large barn door open in the evenings and enjoyed the sounds of innumerable birds calling and animals scuffling in the woods outside. But here I was – on my own, already worrying about the night to come. I settled myself in as best I could indoors then did a small amount of work on Edward Thomas, sitting at the kitchen table. As evening fell I was already beginning to regret my sought-after solitude.

On that first night, when the wood had become a hutch of darkness, I locked the big barn door, ate some supper and went to bed. A piercing light shone directly onto my pillow. I shifted uneasily. It wasn't a moonbeam – far too thin for that. It seemed to find me out, even when I turned on my side. I'd have to sort out some curtains in the morning; meanwhile I got very little sleep and woke un-refreshed.

In the morning, fortified by coffee, I found that the skylights were out of reach even when I was standing on a chair and that there was no ladder anywhere on the premises. I could see no way of making my bedroom private. I must accept it, and make the best of it. I had twenty-seven days to go and a large piece of work I needed to complete. I would spend the mornings writing, then tire myself out so thoroughly with afternoon cliff-walks that nothing – not even this disconcerting light – would keep me awake after going to bed.

CHAPTER THREE: CRISIS

The days were warm and irrelevant. Each day I was unable to forget the coming ordeal, even though I enjoyed my walks and even though I succeeded in maintaining a steady routine of work. Each evening I tried to read or watch television, but sat bewildered by the sensation that I was in a boat rocked by light pouring in through the top of the barn. The walls swayed sickeningly. Each night, below my duvet, I cowered under the searching beam. There was no let-up, no release. Here's a fragment of verse I wrote at the time:

> *The barn rocks like a boat at sea;*
> > *but what pours through the skylight?*
>
> *If it were the moon it would be more diffuse;*
> > *I would feel bathed and blessed.*
>
> *If it were the moon I would sense its tug,*
> > *but not this sickening sway.*
>
> *It probes, it probes, it probes —*
> > *toxic, invasive. I'm defiled.*

I had become convinced that the light must be shining from the road above; and I had come up with an explanation that made sense. It was a man with a torch, standing on the road above the barn; he could see me sweating under the duvet. He wasn't a murderer, though there had been a murder in this valley a few years earlier. He wasn't a rapist or a burglar – if he were one of these, he would surely have broken in and been making noises downstairs? No, his object was nothing less than the possession of my mind and retrieval of my secrets. His beam of torchlight reached into my thoughts. It was piercing like a laser; it sorted through the contents of my brain as if they were emails in my inbox.

Martin (as well as my counsellor) had foreseen that I'd need support while I was away from home and I did call him on the phone from the village regularly. It was hard, though, to explain how very real my fear was, or to feel other than annoyed when he pooh-poohed it. After nearly three weeks of struggling to overcome my embarrassment at asking for help I finally called the police. A young and friendly sergeant turned up to inspect the premises. He agreed that the layout was ideal for a peeping Tom and gave thin reassurances. He suggested putting a piece of cotton across the space where I believed the Torch Man to be standing all night: if it was disturbed in the morning this might mean something... except that a fox could also disturb a piece of cotton. I felt he was laughing at me but rigged up the cotton all the same.

CHAPTER THREE: CRISIS

That night I moved the bed so it faced the other way. The light swayed on the wall as the Torch Man adjusted his position. It was then that I became convinced the Torch Man had been hired by College with the express intention of driving me to distraction. They wanted me out of my job. They were sick of me. They had somehow worked out where my holiday house was and had sent a specially trained spy to look into my brain with his laser beam and reduce me to madness.

That night my terror reached its peak. I tried lying in bed with a screen of pillows propped all round my head to prevent the penetration of the beam. This seemed to madden the Torch Man who walked up and down the path above, angling his light so that it reached me over the top of the pillows. Sweating and shivering with fear I went down into the kitchen and retrieved the largest bin liners I could find. With some Sellotape I managed at long last to rig up a rudimentary blind across the appropriate skylight. I slept fitfully, aware that light was shining in round the edges of the bin liners.

Only a week to go. The kind sergeant returned; we inspected the piece of cotton together and agreed it had not been moved. We sat outside and drank tea while he explained why he'd come back to see me. He'd been looking at maps, working out coordinates, and had realised that the light I was seeing must be Jupiter shining strongly and directly across the fields from the sea. I cross-questioned him, an immense feeling of grateful relief welling up in me. *So it's the same old story, then: a lone woman ravished by God?* We laughed uncomfortably.

How ironic that I had believed Nature would provide me with an escape from my turmoil. Even now I feel bitter about that. I had gone on my working holiday carrying with me the precepts of Richard Mabey's great book, *Nature Cure*. I had gone, moreover, to write about Edward Thomas, whose Nature philosophy now seemed very empty. What had happened to me for four weeks, night after night? I'd been terrorised by a planet and now it was time to go home.

Chapter Four:
The Long Haul

Spring 2010 is here but I scarcely notice what's going on in the garden and feel out of touch with the natural world. I live in a kind of bubble – not listening to the news on the radio, not reading the newspapers, not hearing conversations over lunch. I would call it absent-mindedness but that seems too neutral a phrase. My biggest concern is that I feel my tutorials are less incisive than usual. I'm going through a period of mixed mood again, with disturbed sleep and variable emotions. It's difficult to work out what's happening from the double graph. I'd prefer to talk to someone.

Depression

I take more than 60 mins to fall asleep more than half the time

I awaken at least one hour before I need to and can't go back to sleep

I feel sad nearly all of the time

DIARY OF A BIPOLAR EXPLORER

Most of the time I struggle to focus my attention and make decisions

I think almost constantly about major and minor defects in myself

I feel life is empty and wonder if it's worth living

I am often unable to respond to questions without extreme effort

At times I am unable to stay seated and need to pace around

How is my sleep pattern going?

"Sleep that knits up the ravelled sleeve of care" – where's it gone? I look for it under every shadow of every wall, and in every corner.

What would help to get my sleep back?

"It's gone like the summer, gone like the snow" (Leonard Cohen).

What does the sadness feel like?

Acid rain.

What helps with focusing attention?

Attention to what, focus on what? Work of all kinds is impossible. Songs help, especially by Bob Dylan. So do poems

— not on the page but said aloud. (In the middle of the night, when there's been no sleep for a long time, the focus is sharpest.)

What defects do I notice in myself?

As this will keep us here all day I decline to answer.

Why does it take a long time to respond to questions?

I don't hear them or they're hard; they don't have answers: Why does "ravelled" mean the same as "unravelled"?

Why do I get so tired?

Why is everything so tiring?

Describe something that would make life worth living.

Being able to talk to Sally on the phone while looking at the pear-tree.

Why do I pace around?

To find somewhere else, away from myself, to be.

Mania

I feel happier or more cheerful than usual most of the time

I feel more self-confident than usual most of the time

I frequently need less sleep than usual

I frequently talk more than usual

I have frequently been more active than usual

*

What they don't ask is how I can be sad nearly all of the time in my answer to one questionnaire, and happier than usual most of the time in my answer to another. If they did, I would have to give two answers because they sent me two questionnaires:

1) There's no contradiction.

2) "Do I contradict myself? Very well then, I contradict myself." (Walt Whitman)

Is it good to feel so self-confident, to talk so often?

Don't knock it! I'm unusually large. I contain innumerable multitudes (Whitman again).

How many times have I missed my meds this week?

As many times as necessary.

Sum up – say how it's going, generally.

It's going. Still going.

May 2010: Friendship

I've met up with a friend who suffers from Bipolar Disorder. It's comforting to share tips about how we deal with it. He suffers from it much more severely than I do. He's been in and out of hospital because of psychotic episodes. As a result, he's finding it difficult to hold down a job. A brilliant researcher and a much-loved tutor, he deserves better treatment than he gets in this great collegiate university, where attitudes to mental illness are sometimes unsympathetic. As a temporary lecturer he's treated very poorly, with no help from Occupational Health. Shunted from one short-term badly paid teaching post to another he has no chance of being research-active and of being appointed permanently. He's exhausted, depressed most of the time and only takes sick leave when he absolutely must. There are mechanisms for colleges to make reasonable adjustments in view of disability but these are often ignored. Colleges are in danger of behaving like little fiefdoms. They can kid themselves that they are following their duty of care when they are not equipped to do so. Some of them until recent years may have been under-informed about legislation concerning mental health and about necessary provision for those with disabilities.

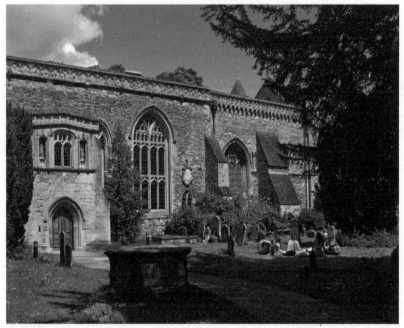

Library Garden, St Edmund Hall (photo by Christopher Cornwell)

June 2010: Mixed mood

Long summer days teaching. The Library Garden in college is at its most lovely in the sun, with students reading among gravestones or lounging in the grass and butterflies flitting among the bushes. I stay up late working. My mixed moods go on much the same; I'm medicated but I don't want to take lithium which inevitably produces weight gain. I fill in the questionnaires dutifully and check in with my consultant to look at the graph.

Chapter Four: The Long Haul

Depression

I take more than 60 mins to fall asleep more than half the time

I awaken at least one hour before I need to and can't go back to sleep

I feel sad nearly all of the time

Most of the time I struggle to focus my attention and make decisions

I think almost constantly about major and minor defects in myself

I feel life is empty and wonder if it's worth living

I am often unable to respond to questions without extreme effort

At times I am unable to stay seated and need to pace around

My mind is turning into a questionnaire. I'm split between questions and answers.

Do I eat more when I feel depressed?

Yes, I find myself eating for England. It feels as though something is compelling me; something driving me on. I'm a human hoover.

What is the connection between sadness and hunger?

Ask the starving millions.

No, the connection for me.

As far as I'm concerned, it's always been there, ever since I was a child. Both are forms of deprivation that nothing can comfort.

What happens when I diet?

Four times in my life I've inflated like a barrage balloon then shrunk by as much as five stone. It's not what they call yo-yo dieting; more like being gripped for years by an obsession then letting go.

And what about alcohol?

That's the same sort of problem, but worse because alcohol is antisocial. However, I've not had any alcohol since September 2002.

Moderation in all things is good, especially if you are bipolar.

Moderation is a word I don't understand. If I were moderate, would I be in this clinic, would I have been filling in questionnaires week after week? Give me the medication that makes me moderate and you can discharge me.

CHAPTER FOUR: THE LONG HAUL

Mania

I often feel happier or more cheerful than usual
I often feel more self-confident than usual
I often need less sleep than usual
I frequently talk more than is usual
I have frequently been more active than usual

*

How can I be feeling sad nearly all of the time and yet happier and more cheerful than usual?

There's no contradiction: I could be feeling sad all the time. That's a viable option and my usual state.

Am I having a period of "mixed mood"?

You tell me, it looks like it from my answers to your questionnaires.

What do I mean by being more "active" than usual?

Thinking more quickly, writing a lot, pacing around the house, talking very fast, taking on unnecessary work, signing up to extra-curricular activities.

What am I finding most difficult?

Holding down a full-time job while being a mum.

October 2010: Mixed mood contd.

I've noticed how manic episodes in my life seem to coincide with the rhythms of the academic year, September being a relatively quiet period when I can concentrate and get some serious academic research done. The symptoms seem to set in as October comes, with the change in light reminding me of dad's death – and this happens exactly as the hothouse atmosphere of the term takes grip. It's always a change in sleep patterns that indicates I'm unwell.

Depression

I take more than 60 minutes to fall asleep, more than half the time

I awaken at least one hour before I need to, and can't go back to sleep

I sleep no longer than 7-8 hours a night without napping during the day.

I feel sad more than half the time

I eat much less than usual and only with personal effort

I have not had a change in my weight

I get tired more easily than usual

There is no change from usual in how interested I am in other people or activities

110

Chapter Four: The Long Haul

Most of the time I struggle to focus my attention or to make decisions

I largely believe that I cause problems for others

I do not think of suicide or death

*

What would help with focus?

Living outside my head.

Why is that so difficult?

There is no outside.

Don't forget the importance of a regular pattern of sleep.

Why is sleep so helpful? We don't know what it does.

We know for sure it's the main thing.

Tell me about it.

What would help, with the sleeping?

Valium; being less worried; swimming, walking, writing; listening to folk songs; living and working somewhere less pressured than Oxford.

Have I ever heard "voices" (i.e. people speaking who were not really present)?

Diary of a Bipolar Explorer

I hear them all the time but I know they're inside my head. None of them break cover into the real world.

We need to check that I never think of suicide or death.

Well, I think of death all the time, lots of deaths – but not my own. I couldn't commit suicide.

Why not?

Because I have a husband and a daughter. It wouldn't be fair on them.

Mania

I feel happier or more cheerful than usual most of the time
I feel more self-confident than usual most of the time
I frequently need less sleep than usual
I frequently talk more than usual
I have frequently been more active than usual

*

In what way have I been more "active" lately?

More driven, more frenzied, and it's all in my head.

What does that feel like?

Caffeine overdose, wasps in a tin; an allergy with no

antidote, an immense recent sting; a laser-beam dancing like a strobe, strip-lights in a hospital flickering; an incessant rhyme scheme with no syntax, lyrics from three songs mixed and melding; everything associated or interconnected in a vast enjoyable pattern with a missing key; waves cresting in time with the undertow; a metallic tunnel and the thoughts bounce on floor wall ceiling but some fly right out into the sunshine and no way to follow.

Why do I feel so tired?

Wouldn't you if your brain was such a happening place?

November 2010: Demonstrations

There's been a major student demonstration in Central London to protest against the raising of student fees and cuts in government funding for universities. Here I am, a member of the establishment and entirely on the students' side. Tertiary education is under pressure; we academics are selling out against our own will to a corporate mentality. How can I as a tutor avoid the feeling that tutorials are becoming a financial transaction and how will this affect my interaction with students? Anger is mounting within the universities; it looks as though the Humanities will suffer most. We could all do without this.

DIARY OF A BIPOLAR EXPLORER

March 2011: Measures

"Stress" is a word so devalued through overuse by pampered members of the middle class that it's almost useless, almost meaningless, especially in the west. How dare we use this word so often and thus traduce the suffering of millions? The average nurse working a shift in A&E goes through more stress in one night than I'll ever know. Yet here am I, with an illness that will show at the slightest sign of disturbance. I'm held in thrall by a glaring absence: let's call it proportion, or experience. Where are others in this anatomy of stress? If I suffered more I might *feel* I suffer less. And yet my illness is real enough. Should we measure what my "needs" are by some objective set of norms or abandon all measures and take my word for it? Where am I, the patient, in this climate of assessment? Must I, as a subject, submit to scrutiny, to this constant scientific charting of my distress? Am I a yardstick? "Reason not the need; our basest beggars /Are in the poorest things superfluous." So raged the pampered King Lear, before he learnt what it was to be a beggar, live in a hovel, and descend into madness. Poor old man. He certainly knew stress.

CHAPTER FOUR: THE LONG HAUL

Spring 2011: Something wicked this way comes

I'm back at home recuperating after a serious neurological episode which landed me in hospital for a week and from which it's taking a long time to recover. The experience was profoundly shocking. *"By the pricking of my thumbs/ Something wicked this way comes."* That's exactly how it started – with a strange insistent prickly feeling in one finger of my left hand which got hotter and more painful as it spread into all four fingers and thumb. I couldn't type. I could pick things up with the hand but only very clumsily.

The first symptoms appeared at the height of a period of anxiety in College. I had been fighting for the rights of a member of staff who had been, as I saw it, roughly treated; and my holiday in Borrowdale had been dominated by emails passing to and fro in a dispute which was getting nowhere. At first I connected the symptoms with anxiety; I even thought I might be imagining them. After a week, with the situation worsening, I knew something serious was afoot. Back in Oxford my GP made immediate contact with the hospital to set up an appointment. "I don't know what it is," she said, shaking her head, "something neurological." I was scared; went home to take things easy.

Diary of a Bipolar Explorer

The initial symptoms were followed by numbness spreading up my left arm, then down my left leg. Just as I thought it was going to stop, the whole process started up on the right hand side of my body, following an identical pattern – first in the fingers, hot and prickly, then down into the legs, cold and numb. Soon the numbness was so acute I was finding it difficult to coordinate my movements. My alarm was now reaching an extreme pitch, with sleepless nights following as a consequence.

At the hospital I was shown into a tiny room by a kind secretary. Martin came with me to help me walk. The Consultant neurologist, a world expert in Multiple Sclerosis, examined me. I couldn't balance enough to walk in a straight line; he did some other tests and said he would keep a watching brief until I'd had an MRI. He sounded unhurried but I was so scared by the appointment that I needed a glass of water. He was gentle and comforting. He observed that I seemed acutely stressed. When I expressed my fear of MS and death he told me that this was not an immediate prospect. In the loo afterwards I threw up.

Two days later I couldn't get my eyes to focus and was admitted to the Neurology ward in the John Radcliffe with an urgent request for a CAT scan and an MRI. Martin came with me. On the way from the lift to the ward I saw signs saying "DOMESTIC WASTE ONLY" and was back in the psychiatric ward in Leeds. White lights glared at me, white walls caged me. There were no pictures; no flowers were allowed to be brought by visitors because of the danger of spreading germs. My bed looked out on a cemetery. Everything was cold and smelled of antiseptic.

I had a throbbing pain at the back of my head and my fingers were so hot and prickly that I was given codeine to help control the pain. They ran test after test. I was by now unable to walk at all and was wheeled round in a wheelchair to get me to my various tests. When I went to the loo a nurse helped me. I had lost my privacy and dignity. I felt I was old before my time.

The brain scan revealed a lesion at the base of my brain, just where it meets the top of the spine. This explained the pain and also why all parts of my body and my vision were affected. That is the spot where all the nerves come together. There were two tiny lesions elsewhere in the brain but nowhere on my spine. This meant that the Multiple Sclerosis was in its very early stages, if MS it was. I was in the clear as regards tumours and the doctors' initial worries about a possible breast-cancer were quickly allayed. I was therefore facing a possible MS diagnosis and awaiting a lumbar puncture.

Diary of a Bipolar Explorer

On the ward I soon understood that I was in among people who had very severe symptoms of MS or worse. Everyone admitted to the ward was there to undergo an operation; I was the only one admitted for tests only. The woman opposite had suffered a massive brain haemorrhage. During my time there she underwent an operation to pin her brain together with twenty pins. I saw her surrounded by joyful children afterwards and rapidly re-calibrated my own condition as minor. All the same, it was terrifying to be in the company of people suffering from serious MS symptoms and to know that one day I might be in that position. I was haunted by the memory of seeing a friend with MS in the last months of her life, lying a vegetable on her bed, able only to move her lips – and those with difficulty.

During the day all was relatively stable so far as my mood disorder went. I got to know the nurses and fellow patients; I enjoyed the camaraderie. I had my favourites among the doctors who daily made their rounds. I was visited in hospital by Martin, my step-daughter Fiona and by Emma on the eve of her GCSE in history. She looked so small, so defenceless and scared as she sat on the edge of the bed and tried to make small talk.

CHAPTER FOUR: THE LONG HAUL

At night the lights tormented me. Underfunding can be the only legitimate explanation for the glare of strip-lighting on the wards as nurses make their night rounds, intermittently called to bedsides by patients pressing loud alarms. Gradually the sleeplessness got to me, a kind of torture. Images of the First World War came back to haunt me. I found myself on the verge of another psychotic episode, but thankfully the period of hallucination was brief.

A lumbar puncture didn't confirm MS and when I was discharged from hospital it was with an ambiguous diagnosis. I left having learned a lot about how the brain functions and with a renewed respect for all the doctors and nurses who do such good work in their daily lives. I've also learned two further things. Firstly, that there is a great deal more sympathy for a physical disease like MS than there is for a mental one like Bipolar Disorder. In the Psychiatric Wing in Leeds I was visited by Martin and a friend wrote to me there. In hospital in Oxford I had three visitors and was surrounded by cards, gifts, messages of support from friends, colleagues, family. Everyone knew this was serious. MS is a serious condition and I don't want to diminish that fact; but then so too is BD. There appears to be a double standard in our culture which dictates that illness which can be seen is somehow more "real", more worthy of respect and acknowledgement, than illness which is invisible. My consultant psychiatrist once said of his patients, "If they were in a wheelchair, their employers would be rolling out the ramps for them. As it is they get zero help." Gerard Manley Hopkins knew a thing or two about all kinds of suffering and I think of his words often: "Hold them cheap/ May who ne'er hung there."

The second thing I've learned is that just as there's a double standard in society about mind and body, so in western medicine there's a kind of blindness to the way symptoms interconnect. Throughout my treatment for suspected MS I've been seen by a number of different doctors, all of whom have commented on the role that my Bipolar Disorder played in exacerbating the stress of hospital visits etc. But what of the possibility that BD and MS are both manifestations of a single problem? At no stage until I suggested it has anyone thought to look at me holistically as a single person with the same mind, the same body. I've been from neurology to psychiatry looking for an answer to the basic question, "How am I ill and what causes this?" I shall always trust a pricking in my thumb to tell me that something wicked this way comes. It doesn't matter to me whether we classify the "something wicked" as physical or mental; the two are inseparable.

CHAPTER FOUR: THE LONG HAUL

August-September 2011: Recovery

Slowly, bit by bit, I'm becoming able to walk normally again and the use of my hands is gradually returning. I've taught myself to use a voice-recognition device on my computer. This is enabling me to continue the work on my book about the Wordsworths, which had been interrupted by illness. In the early summer we moved into the cottage at Cornwall which we've just bought as a second home and we've been having a long period of relaxation living healthily and settling into the Roseland, familiar to us from many Easter holidays in this very cottage. August has been spent with my family, walking and gardening. The steady rhythm of walking is good for mental and physical health. Daily trips to the sea have filled me with energy; my excess weight has dropped off and now, in mid-September, I feel well. I've been taking all the supplements recommended for MS and this seems to be doing the trick. A month on my own – reading, writing, thinking, and walking – will surely complete my recovery.

October 2011: A tragic death

Sabbatical leave is darkened by the death of a former student, at more or less the same age as my sister and from the same cause – cancer. She was a gifted Romanticist:

the sad news sends a huge shock through the scholarly community. I had seen her very recently and known she was sick, but not realised that her condition was terminal. Guilt is a normal reaction to death: I find myself thinking about what I could have done had I known. My depression is mild this time, but I'm again experiencing the recurring pattern of reactive illness that comes whenever someone I know dies, prompting memories of deaths in my own family. I remember her as a student and try to draw inspiration from her personality and successful career.

February 2012: The poetry workshop

I've been running writing workshops for several years now – the students drop in to my room in College bringing their latest work. This provides a steady creative rhythm.

The workshop

We come looking for nothing more
than what we find, listening in turn
to each other read.

There's something of magic ritual
in the handing-out of pages,
the agreement of an order.

122

Chapter Four: The Long Haul

There's something of reverence
in our stillness, heads bent
over the writing, our attention.

If there's a break in concentration,
it's only a pause for reflection,
before the comments -

like a long draught to one who thirsts,
or a walk on the moors in the high wind
to one who's trapped and forsaken.

The whole week turns on this.

2012: A quiet year

Aside from a trip to York for Jane's memorial service in the Minster (a grand and beautiful occasion) this has been a quiet year of scholarship, bringing my book on the Wordsworths to completion. My own experience of recovery through nature's healing has spurred me on to revise the book with bereavement and healing as its central themes. I've become preoccupied by Lewis Hyde's great book, *The Gift*, in which the value of reciprocal and communal creativity is celebrated. His argument is finding its way into my writing. I begin to understand why I'm so interested in my students' creativity and why this brings me greater rewards than my normal focus on their academic work. There are two economies that run alongside each other in relation to my students: one involves their formal education, for which as an academic I'm paid. The other involves overseeing and encouraging their creative life: this is voluntary work, and immensely appreciated by them. The two economies must coexist, in my experience, for my job to be fulfilling. This idea of a double economy seems to me to be the essence of what it is to be a teacher; it's also crucial I think to most writers because it's what makes culture thrive. Writers must find ways of honouring this double economy if their work is to make a valuable contribution.

With all this at the forefront of my mind I've persuaded College to let me put together a coherent publicity campaign for "Writing at the Hall", so as to foster our ongoing creative community; and over the summer I've compiled a Directory of all the writers who read English at the college. This work has been taxing; I'm corresponding with my former pupils and learning how to create and load copy into a website. Gradually the Directory is taking shape. Has there been an element of hypomania in all this activity? Possibly, but if it's not followed by the usual slump into depression I'll begin to feel that I'm on an even keel. My academic duties are manageable and Michaelmas Term looks set to go smoothly.

October 2012: Post-Traumatic Stress Disorder

Why does a bright light shining in the darkness make me shudder? Why does the image of a camera make me feel anxious? Why are eyes and images of eyes such powerful signifiers and why do they appear everywhere in my poems? Some people have inescapable visual memories: it seems that I'm one of them. I'm bothered by various recurring visual images and have been referred for assessment to the Warneford, where I've received a diagnosis of Post-Traumatic Stress Disorder. The visual images that I find distressing are easily traced back to the psychotic episode in Leeds and to subsequent episodes involving paranoid delusions – including the Torch Man and the theft of my confidential dossier in 2008. I'm surprised at the powerful hold that these triggers have on my moods after so many years. We've also discovered a trigger that originated the day of Sally's death, when I saw her unclosed staring eyes as she lay dead. The morbid nature of my fascination with eyes scares and repels me.

Diary of a Bipolar Explorer

I've become involved in a fascinating research project which trials an innovative method for helping the brain to re-process traumatic material. I'm being taught how to re-visit traumatic memories, how to picture them differently as I re-approach them, and how to run through an entire scenario as if from a different perspective, supplying different visual details. The exercises are in effect training my mind in narratology as well as in understanding the triggers that induce distress. Technically, I'm finding ways of causing new neural pathways to open up in my brain so that obsessional thought-patterns associated with trauma can be replaced with calming ones that won't upset me. I'm working with two extremely clever women whose skill and camaraderie help me to understand much of the traumatic content of distressing episodes in the past. I find temporary fulfilment in the process of re-mapping and the whole experience gives me much food for thought. I'm not sure how much of what I value in this is to do with the pleasure of interaction – a kind of talking cure – and how much to do with the mechanics of narration, but the process certainly helps.

At Christmas, relaxed in Cornwall with the family, I celebrate ten years of abstinence from alcohol by raising a glass of wine to the health of all and drinking it!

CHAPTER FOUR: THE LONG HAUL

February 2013: A new community

I'm bringing together a large community of writers to celebrate writing. We've launched an online resource, the Hall Writers' Forum, in which I've found a group of people who share my interests. I've entered a new absorbing world. Having had no experience of such things before I'm surprised by how quickly I've taken to the activity of posting and reading posts. I don't anticipate there being any serious dangers in this for myself, though some warning signs may be there.

June 2013: Relapse

Something wicked this way comes. It's back – the pricking in my fingers which soon becomes hot pain; the numbness spreading up my arm. The relapse has been brought on by a period of marking in Finals, when I've been using my fingers to hold a pen rather than to type. I sympathise with the poor finalists, who have to do this day after day under considerably greater stress than I have been. With the illness recurring, I've assessed the risks of continuing to work while experiencing the double difficulties of BD and MS. I've announced my retirement; I've given away books to my students; I've begun the process of clearing my room…

But it's a false alarm – the symptoms abate. I'm left with some difficulties in College arising from all this and with my book on the Wordsworths to see through the press. A warm breeze blows into the kitchen of our cottage in Cornwall where I sit reading proofs. I'm under deadline pressure yet full of relief at my recovery. I'll need to learn to live with these kinds of relapse if I do have MS, but no-one is giving me a definitive diagnosis. I keep watch.

August 2013: Scotland

My book *William and Dorothy Wordsworth: All in Each Other* was published just before we left for a family holiday in Scotland, so there's been much rejoicing. The holiday – which began with a hectic week at the Edinburgh festival before we wound on to the Highlands – was a rejuvenating success and we've ended up in Grasmere.

I hear the news of Seamus Heaney's death while standing in the museum at Dove Cottage: an appropriate setting, given his connection with the place and with Wordsworth. I'm deeply saddened, as are the staff there. One of them gives me a hug. On the way back to Oxford in the car, listening to the radio as it repeats the shocking news over and over again, I weep for the loss of such a great man and so suddenly. But the sadness can't tip me into depression. I'm on an even keel, buoyed up by the holiday and my book.

January 2014: Where have all the flowers gone?

Pete Seeger has died, so it's like someone has switched off the sun. I cannot imagine the house where I grew up without his songs. Unlike Bob Dylan, who divided us – our parents rushing in to turn the volume down – Pete's voice was welcome all day long, from the kitchen to the attic: every door ajar, everyone listening as they did their cooking, homework, marking. He stopped us in our tracks to sing of war, injustice, oppression, in piercing words never to be forgotten. His ballads held the line, piecing the truth together. In the summer, with all the windows open, his melodies filled the garden; he married folk to protest and made them last for ever. Not once did we see his optimism waver. I'm here in Oxford when I learn he's died, but my thoughts are in our house in Leeds as grief grips hard – five decades since the Sixties suddenly un-spooling. Over the phone, family members mutter timid useless consolations and are agreed: with Pete Seeger gone, the world's a gutted candle, a broken heart.

DIARY OF A BIPOLAR EXPLORER

May 2014: Dependency

When I log in to the Hall Writers' Forum I have the strange illusion of being inside a parallel world. It's like a rickety old house with an attic and a cellar. The attic is the section open to public view and is separated from the section reserved for members only, which I associate with a dusty cellar. Of course I know I'm online and this is just a virtual community; yet the sense of inhabiting a physical place is very strong. I've also come to think of the Forum as corresponding in a metaphorical way to the human psyche as Freud understood it, with a supervening ego upstairs and an unconscious downstairs. All the preparatory work, all the messy stuff, gets posted below in the reserved section, invisible to the prying eyes of strangers. All the polished work gets posted upstairs – part of the college's public face, its outreach activities attracting attention. The sense of a psyche split across the middle is almost as palpable as the spatial sense of moving around within a house. I'm beginning to inhabit the Forum as if it were myself – or perhaps I should put that the other way round? The Forum is beginning to inhabit me. Gaston Bachelard, who wrote beautifully in *The Poetics of Space* about how actual places become internalised, would have a field-day with the implications of this kind of imagining.

130

Chapter Four: The Long Haul

September 2014: The dangers of social media

Oh how I'm coming to hate Facebook, its shiny world of trivia! There've been numerous studies of the damaging effects of social media on the fabric of human lives and relationships, but I don't need these to tell me that over-use can lead rapidly to feelings of loneliness, dependency, loss of self-respect and even serious addiction. Facebook, the most widely used and successful of the available social media, is said by some researchers to be gradually losing its appeal to users. I've tried it for less than a year and during that time I've become damagingly addicted to the rewards of self-reassurance which a circle of supportive friends seem to provide. Like many Facebook users I've gathered together a much larger circle of so-called friends than was necessary and have often been saddened not to receive the kind of self-validation that I've come to expect and crave from such a sizeable group. The number of "likes" and "shares" which I get each day has become important to me. I resemble a performing animal, waking up each morning to decide what I'll post for my 500 or so "friends". I dislike my Facebook self so strongly that I have to leave. I won't regret it. From now on I will make friends only in the real world. I will also follow the advice of Socrates, as far as this is possible: "Be slow to fall into friendship, but when you are in, continue firm and constant."

Diary of a Bipolar Explorer

November 2014: Addiction

Vast tracts of time disappear as I sit reading posts on the Forum. The time feels alive while it's happening, but wasted and dead almost as soon as it's gone. I keep involved because interactions are engaging and worthwhile. I learn so much. I know very few of the people who post there but they *feel* like friends – real friends, as distinct from some of the fakery that happens on Facebook. Does this medium offer an escape from my responsibilities and the drudgery of life? I think so. I've been doing less about the house since the neurological episode and almost none since I discovered social media. I've almost lost the ability to sit and read a book and to concentrate on academic writing. I'm failing to make genuine contact with colleagues or to sustain real relationships at home. I'm neglecting my family. During the working week everything that happens in my teaching is squeezed into the spaces between Forum posts. At weekends I can spend whole days posting material, thinking about it, responding. It has become an alternative space in which to live. Enthusiasm has shaded into addiction.

CHAPTER FOUR: THE LONG HAUL

April-May 2015: Campaigning

The Campaign to elect the Nigerian writer Wole Soyinka as our next Oxford Professor of Poetry is no mean undertaking. I'm working like a Trojan to lead it and make it a success. There have been many missions in my life but never one on which I've concentrated with such driven intensity. I'm meant to be reading Finals dissertations yet every minute of every day is taken up with emails and Forum posts. (The Hall Writers' Forum is Campaign Headquarters.) To bring the election off successfully would be a triumph for the University. I got into this almost by accident through a personal family connection with Soyinka. Now the whole process feels almost inevitable, as though I'm turning into my campaigning mother. They say that Bipolar Disorder sometimes produces delusions of grandeur. Am I in danger of these? An ambition to transform poetry at Oxford is the reason for this Campaign yet there are personal investments: the wish to succeed, to have influence, and the need to make a connection with my birthplace Uganda by contact with this Nigerian writer who's a family friend.

I've been in a state of agitation throughout the Easter vacation and have only just managed to complete my marking as term comes. The results of the UK General Election cast an almighty pall over the beginning of the summer term.

June 2015: The campaign continues

Why is it so difficult to persuade the University's graduate electorate that Oxford should acknowledge achievements and contributions made by a great writer who addresses the burning issues – a writer who has been imprisoned, who has championed reformist ideals, and whose work has been honoured with a Nobel Prize? Things have turned ugly in the press and the rigmarole for voting is in urgent need of reform because the powerful forces of British insularity have taken grip. The move to elect Soyinka as our next Oxford Professor of Poetry has become an international grass roots campaign. The stress is almost overwhelming – long work stretching into the night; a little hammer going in my brain all day; a little bird in my chest beating its wings angrily. I'm in what's called a "mixed episode", simultaneously depressed and elated.

Chapter Four: The Long Haul

July 2015: Failure and disappointment

We failed. The disappointment is overwhelming. I have no words to express the disgust I feel towards a certain celebrity who has helped to bring about the results. It's hard not to see this as the defeat of a distinguished African by the petty forces of localism; but Soyinka has accepted the outcome with generosity and grace. There's been some coverage of our disappointment in the press. I'm recuperating slowly, cursing the establishment while trying to focus on academic work. I've written a long opinion piece, published in the *Times Higher,* protesting against the pathetic electoral process and the exclusion of students from the right to vote.

Writing a plenary lecture for the upcoming Wordsworth Conference distracts me from the anti-climax. But I ward off depression in the wrong way, drinking alcohol instead of walking. The long awaited publication of my book of poems, *Earth's Almanac*, goes by almost unnoticed in the aftermath of the election.

August 2015: A long tired summer

At our cottage in Cornwall I'm unable to enjoy the beautiful countryside that surrounds me, unable even to take my favourite walk from the cottage to the beach. Exhaustion makes it impossible to do more than about fifteen minutes of work at a time and I find that even small amounts of reading make matters worse. The summer is going by in a kind of haze; I listen to a great deal of British folk music and work desultorily. Over and over I play Dick Gaughan's version of a great socialist song by Leon Rosselsson, "World turned upside down". I write my own words to the tune of it, telling the story of Soyinka's defeat. This poem will be published in a book I'm co-editing about the failed election. I try to edit Edward Thomas's *In Pursuit of Spring* but am able to do only a kind of hackwork job on his most beautiful book. Completion of this will have to be postponed.

September, my favourite month, is about to start. I'm on my own in this cottage. I can't face the journey north to Leeds to see my mum, who has had a fall and broken her ankle. When I eventually go (with Martin and Emma) I cross the threshold with trepidation, remembering the morning of psychosis. But it's right to see her, to touch base. Home again I find comfort in the community of the Hall Writers' Forum, in emails with good friends I've made there and in a new friendship with my sister Gill, who listens to me and talks openly about difficulties in the family. Thoughts of term-time were already worrying me as July turned into August. As September slips away I feel concerned about the stress ahead. Returning to the home of lost causes, I mourn the disappearance of an entire summer.

September 2015: Further thoughts on social media

For patients suffering from Bipolar Disorder, involvement in social media is potentially more damaging than for those who have no disability. There's a danger that it intensifies obsessive activity, exacerbating mood-swings and even triggering episodes. I certainly found Facebook to be destructive. My addiction to the Forum is fundamentally creative. As the person in charge I'm obliged to read all the material that comes in; this gives me a reason (or should that be "pretext"?) for daily interaction. I'm also heavily involved in the content of what's posted because this Forum is a serious medium for exchange and discussion shared by writers whom I deeply respect. Very little trivia appears on the Forum, where the rewards of involvement far outweigh the disadvantages. But it has become a burden, a source of anxiety – even, occasionally, the cause of paranoia.

Diary of a Bipolar Explorer

October 2015: Emma's departure

The horse-chestnut trees are laden with conkers. Normally I would be out looking for their gleam among the fallen leaves around South Park. Taking Emma to Cambridge, unpacking her boxes and seeing her safely settled into a room overlooking the Cam, I feel a combination of excitement and dazed incredulity. How can this moment have arrived so soon? Where have the years gone? Can she really be the same age as the First Year undergraduates I'm about to meet for the first time back in Oxford? Outside, where the punts are turning, a guide is talking loudly in a dreary monotone about the history of her College, Trinity Hall. Ducks are flapping and gliding; we can hear lovers talking as they walk through the passageway under the window. In the corridor I meet another parent carrying a whole load of stuff into the next-door room: his son will be Emma's neighbour. I remember all the many years I've watched parents carrying their children's belongings into my own College. How odd to be at last on the other side of this system of exchange. At least I'll be able to picture her in her own environment as we return this evening to our empty house. She looks small but purposeful and independent as we say goodbye in the front quad – her kiss almost perfunctory, as if she fears being watched by her future friends. I turn to wave goodbye as she pushes the immense wooden gate shut. She doesn't see me waving.

November 2015: Empty nest syndrome

The apples are all gathered in and stored away. Martin is clearing the lawn of fallen leaves as I watch him from the window. There's a calm sense of completion in the scene outside that sits oddly alongside my growing unease. Like all the big biological transitions in life this is not one I could possibly have prepared for. In the gaps between teaching I wander the house aimlessly, conscious of an absence. Not just of a person, but of a whole load of clutter – and of an atmosphere, a way of being. There's no more banter, no more quarrelling about tiny domestic things, no more slamming of my door shut because I'm thought to be playing the wrong music. Emma's bedroom is uncannily tidy: everything she needed she has taken with her, everything she didn't she has cleared away. She has put all her CDs into a disused doll's house, having copied each and every one of them onto her computer before leaving. I don't feel desolate at first, just numb and confused like our cat who winds herself round my feet and whimpers. Gradually the finality of loss makes itself felt and a familiar cloud of depression settles on me. Aside from the fulfilment of my contractual obligations at work I'm struggling to get through each day. I feel much as I did when I had a miscarriage in my late thirties. I try to use the Forum to fill the emptiness but it can't overcome a sense of bereavement.

December 2015: My last admissions exercise

Retirement beckons. I've decided to take it five years early – not for reasons of ill health, but because I'm disillusioned by the increasingly corporate direction in which tertiary education is moving. How strange to think that all the tutorials I've given this term are the last I shall ever give; and that this is the final generation of students I'll help to admit to College. There's something valedictory in all this, in amongst the usual pressure and excitement of interviewing for Admissions.

As Christmas approaches an argument is heating up on the Hall Writers' Forum about whether the statue of Cecil Rhodes at Oriel College should be removed. It's a divisive issue with fierce arguments being conducted in the press. I'm being drawn into the debate, which becomes riskily all-consuming. Should Oriel disown this famous alumnus because of his shameful history? Has that history been misrepresented by students keen to stamp their mark? Is it the job of the establishment to preserve its heritage, no matter how disgraceful? Should the statue come down to loud acclaim from protesters, or should it be turned quietly inward on Oriel College, so that the College can take responsibility for the origins of its wealth? I wander the streets of Oxford, looking at the Colleges and thinking about the history of colonialism that's inscribed in their grand architecture and their endowments. This gives a whole new meaning to the phrase "ivory towers". I feel shame, as I did after the Professor of Poetry election, to belong to an institution with this heritage. As the Forum community becomes more divided my own commitment to removal of the statue deepens. I watch out for a mood-swing in the upward direction as my Forum activity increases.

December 2016: A ritual

Every Christmas I read *Elegies*, Douglas Dunn's miraculous collection of poems about the death of his wife from cancer. Doing this is my way of marking Sally's death and reminding myself of the way poetry emerges out of the process of grieving. This year I've also read Max Porter's *Grief is the Thing with Feathers* and been deeply moved. Is it morbid to be so preoccupied with the poetry of grief? I keep going back to Thomas Hardy; his sardonic humour, even in the grimmest of poems about death, is welcome.

Diary of a Bipolar Explorer

January 2016: Sonnets

I'm writing sonnets intensively. The process reminds me of writing my first collection *Ginnel*. These are sonnets about the Wordsworths in 1802, and they have me revisiting work I did for my book *William and Dorothy Wordsworth: All in Each Other*. It's extraordinary to be entering into the lives of these writers empathetically, using dramatic monologue to voice their thoughts and feelings. As soon as I finish one poem another starts to form in my mind. I feel energised by the activity, perhaps even on the edge of hypomania. I post excessively on the Forum.

February 2016: "Lurkers"

The vocabulary used to describe Forum readers is immensely evocative: "Lurkers". Who would not at the back of their minds associate the word with something sinister? There are so many of them! We can tell they're there by the innumerable footprints they leave – every visit to the Forum gets recorded in a tally. Lurkers are welcome because they give us a sense of purpose. When no-one's posting, when no one responds to what we write, they are quietly reading – or so it seems. But this is somewhat frightening. Are we, the members of this Forum, just performers exposed to the gaze of passive consumers? We're being watched by silent strangers; does this turn us into a kind of spectacle? Whatever we type into the Forum is there forever, a record of what we thought and felt. Is privacy the best option? Is it best to remain detached and reticent? How about posting anonymously?

March 2016: Emoticons

In social media, some communication happens through non-verbal signs such as emoticons. On the Forum, I'm beginning to get a handle on the systems of defence that these involve.

Dear Emoticons,

You arrived late in the game, but you're welcome! How I love you, my little flock of obedient creatures! You make it so easy to be just a bit abrasive, just a little contentious. I can even say something quite outrageous and then ever so slightly un-say it, just by picking out one of your amazing range of tones and postures! Easy as that. One click, and there you are: the reliable ones. No-one could possibly misread you. ☺

Yours unpredictably
LN

DIARY OF A BIPOLAR EXPLORER

April 2016: "Guests"

Am I going a bit mad? Even the Forum's Reserved Section is being visited! At the bottom of the screen it sometimes says "1 guest" alongside my own name. The first time this happened it struck me as impossible – but now it lurks more and more often. Of course I feel a strange kinship with the invisible eye whenever our lurkings coincide – but still I sweat with fear. If it came in twos or threes I would worry less. It's the singularity, the cold malevolent presence of that one and only guest that terrifies me.

May 2016: Bots

I've discovered that many of the lurkers on the Forum are spider robots! I feel curiously resentful, as well as spied upon. The feeling of surveillance from the web is alarmingly strong and pervasive.

> *Dear Sogou Web Spider, Yahoo Help Us Slurp, Drupal Org, Googlebot, Bingbot, Yahoobot, Dotbot, Colwis Spider Nutch and Firefox Mutant Daum,*
>
> *Hello! It's my turn to keep the day-watch – and yes, the night-watch too. As nothing else is happening on the Forum, I've been watching you. It's no clearer to*

me now than it was last time what you're doing in this place – all day, all night, on and off, off and on, on and off when so little is happening...when, to be frank, it's more or less a morgue in here. Oh, what good company you make! What fine lines you thread when no one else is around. How visible and welcome you are to me in my Invisible Spy Chamber observing you. Are you spinning your web? Are you patrolling? Or are you simply watching, waiting, and collecting data? I'm told there's a Huge World of Interconnected Knowledge Out There and that you help to bring it all together. That's nice! Meanwhile the dust is gathering. I can just make out the soft tippety-tap of your feet as you crawl the empty corridors...and if I hold very still I can hear you spinning. Make no mistake, I'm keeping tabs on you. Bye for now. I'll hope to catch you later.

Yours
LN

June-July 2016: Brexit

In the burnt fields of Cornwall, nothing but dried-out wasted grain; barley tasteless in the aftermath. Like most of the people I know I'm astounded by the Brexit referendum, which casts a shadow over the summer – but there's solidarity in disgust and this doesn't cause clinical depression. There's something about living half the time in Cornwall that makes a difference to how one sees the results, this being a county that has its own separate identity and culture. It's more or less an independent country. A "leave" vote comes as less of a jolt in this community than it does back in Oxford. *Onen hag oll*. Farmers are content; offcomers count their houses while ageing hippies curse.

August 2016: Room clearance

Outside my room in College the lawn shrinks, brown-edged; the yew-tree almost reaches in, not quite. I've been gradually clearing my books out, carload by carload, and settling them in at home ready for my retirement in October. I've had a recurring dream of falling down the stairs and lying senseless. What does this signify, is it some kind of warning? I step carefully, warily. Today the maintenance team came with a van to transport the main bulk of my possessions, leaving the room denuded: no library, no bric-a-brac; only dust – and spiders, surprised. I haven't scratched my name on the window-pane or under the window-seat but I've left a few things (mainly useful) like mugs, paper-clips, cushions, for the next inhabitant.

Chapter Four: The Long Haul

My friends in Maintenance have stopped me from feeling sad till the very end with all their joshing and banter. Now...well, we're unable to move at home for boxes. In the garden, wind stirs among the apple-trees and the small fruit already fall. Washing flaps and twists on the line; our cat chases a white butterfly; the window rattles in its frame. A climbing rose trails against the pane.

Chapter Five:
Retirement and
Breakdown

The summer's over. October's here and the day of my retirement has come. Conkers gleam among fallen leaves on Old Road; apples fall each day onto our lawn. It's over – I'm no longer a wage-slave. So where's my elation, my sense of release? All I can feel is a sense of being emptied out, depleted. Like Othello, "my occupation's gone." My books are all removed from my room in college and re-housed at home on new bookshelves; my paintings and bric-a-brac have found places too. Still I'm unable to settle.

The college dinner in my honour caused me much anxiety. There was a very kind and generous speech from a colleague and dear friend, but my own speech was an anti-climax. Summaries of what I've done, what I've achieved, seem beside the point in a world where the Brexit vote turned out as it did; and where so many unfinished projects stare me in the face. I see a series of

CHAPTER FIVE: RETIREMENT AND BREAKDOWN

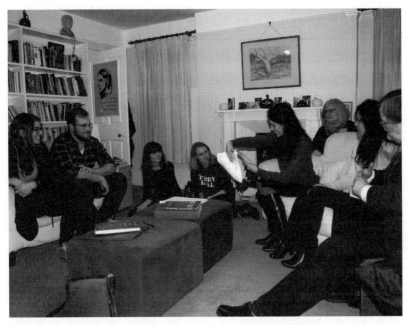

A Wednesday Workshop in my room in college (photo by Claire Hooper)

blank days stretching before me, in which I'll miss my habitual contact with students. There's much work for me to do but I wander desultorily, reading a bit here, a bit there. I can't concentrate.

There's a poem by the American poet James Wright which describes lying lazily in a hammock observing the natural world. It ends abruptly with the sentence, "I have wasted my life". As I look back at vast tracts of time I can't account for I feel the same.

October 2016: That time of year again

Emma has gone off to Cambridge. Term has started up here without me. I wonder will I ever get used to the strange rhythm of her arrivals and departures? Only two academic years left in which to be reminded of the structure which used to hold my life in some kind of order; then it will be over and she'll have left home.

Our rosemary bush is enormously overgrown and visited daily by stray cats. Our own cat is disturbed. All day she wanders distracted about the house – looking for a place to settle, looking for more to eat. As I go downstairs she wraps herself clingingly around my feet. When I hold hard to the handrail, fearing for my life, she reaches up to scratch me. Is she testing me, trying to compete? When I sit on the sofa she comes and sits nearby – but if I try to stroke her she bites. I watch her, she watches me. I've begun to wonder as I wander about if we're as mad as Cowper's "Crazy Kate".

November 2016: Hypomania

What is it that prompts a hypomanic episode? Is it simply a chemical reaction in the body, or are there other explanations? There's some evidence that a narrowly

150

biomedical approach to the illness is inadequate. In this instance I would have a hard time explaining the swing in my mood, one of the most sudden and extreme I've ever experienced. Is it caused mainly by the disruption of retirement? It follows a short spell of low mood and appears to be a reaction to extended discussion on the Forum about Bob Dylan's Nobel Prize. Elated at first by the news of his success, I've gone through a period of complex soul-searching in which the history of this prize – specifically its connection with arms-trading – has become a reason for disapproving of Dylan's eventual acceptance of the honour. I've been looking back on his long career, questioning the shift from protest to rock. Did he sell out to the establishment; have the forces of capitalism trapped him? Will he have the strength of character to appear at the Nobel Prize ceremony and surprise everyone by turning it down? I want him to refuse it (as did Jean-Paul Sartre) even though I'm enormously gratified by the recognition of him as a poet. I'm divided down the middle: my role as a member of the literary establishment is in friction with my love of all that Dylan's idealised image stands for.

There comes a point where intellectual debate won't resolve a moral conundrum that seems to have personal implications. The emotions are hard to manage. I feel extremely overwrought. I listen all day to Dylan's songs. This period of turmoil (together with an emotional meeting with Wole Soyinka and other events in the world) is finally tipping me over the edge.

November 2016: Collapse

Armistice Day. I wander about Headington in a daze, stunned by the victory of Trump and the death of Leonard Cohen. Red and white poppies both seem equally shameful. Now I'm pacing around all the time; smoking and drinking to excess; talking too much and obsessionally; high as a kite but also depressed by recent events. Sleep is impossible. Eventually, realising something is badly wrong, I ring my GP and get an immediate referral to the Warneford team who see me straight away. I am as they put it "elevated". I've caught the mood-swing just in time and am now back in the professionals' care.

November 2016: The confession

Dear Forum Friends,

We've celebrated and questioned Bob Dylan's Nobel Prize; we've watched Trump in his victory; we've lamented Leonard Cohen's death; Now I have my own news. I'm sick. You may have guessed this from the way I've been over-reacting recently. I'm getting the right kind of help and medication. Here's a long post to explain my case-history of bipolarity. Make of it what you will. I hope this explains my over-posting. I hope you'll understand my addiction. I hope you'll bear with me in my long-postponed "outing".

Love, Lucy

I feel raw, as if the whole of my skin had been stripped away. Why this compulsion to confess? My Forum friends are helping me with their feedback but I feel dependent, abject, defence-less. I would not have been able to "confess" like this if the Forum were still open to public view; it's only because we've recently made it private that I felt brave enough to put my thoughts in writing. My posts will only be read by the small group of members who regularly log in. Even so, it's not always that easy to see who's a friend. Sometimes they cluster thickly, sometimes they thin out, like noiseless shadows. I think I know the real friends though. They aren't always the ones who bring good news. The immensity of their insight humbles and astonishes me.

November 2016: The questionnaires return

For years now I've not been bothering to fill in the questionnaires about mood disorder: I felt that my identity had got lost in them. Now, because I'm so sick, they're back, and they provide a useful method of keeping tabs on my moods – useful for the doctors that is; I don't find them directly helpful.

Depression

I take more than 60 minutes to fall asleep, more than half the time
I awaken more than once a night and stay awake for 20 minutes or more, more than half the time
I awaken at least one hour before I need to, and can't go back to sleep
I feel sad more than half the time
There is no change in my usual appetite
I have not had a change in my weight
Most of the time I struggle to focus my attention or to make decisions
There is no change from usual in how interested I am in other people or activities
I largely believe that I cause problems for others
I do not think of suicide or death

Chapter Five: Retirement and Breakdown

*

They want to know about my interest in people and activities. Does it fluctuate? they ask.

There are times when I can scarcely get out of bed. Other times I'm driven and my writing is wholly absorbing.

What does it feel like, what do they both feel like?

Staying in bed is like being sixteen again, hiding from the day. I have no energy, my whole sap is sunk, my life-blood is drained away. Feeling driven is knowing there's one and one thing only to be done and nosing it out. In the day I'm either hunting solitude like it's a drug or I'm gregarious, wanting to throw myself into my activities. Either I'm talking far too much or I'm shutting out people, noises, distraction – moving from room to be on my own, hiding myself away online.

How quickly does it turn from one mood to the other?

It varies. Sometimes they're so close together I can't tell them apart.

Do you think your behaviour is antisocial?

Yes it's antisocial. It's sometimes easier to be with people online.

Why's that?

Absence. There's time to react; you don't have to see emotion in their faces. Everything stills to a hush round writing.

Is it always like that online?

More than in real life. That's why I spend so much of my life there. But then there are the gaps between posts; the waiting to know. Have I or have I not offended?

What does that feel like?

Absence falls from the sky, hollowness folds and holds. Like I'm rubbish, waiting to be sorted for recycling. If I'm re-begot, it will be as John Donne says from "absence, darkness, death - things which are not".

Mania

I often feel happier or more cheerful than usual
I often feel more self-confident than usual
I often need less sleep than usual
I frequently talk more than is usual
I have frequently been more active than usual

*

Is there anything that will help?

I'm not needing help with this.

They remind me of the need for sleep.

I don't need any more sleep than I'm getting; if possible I would like less.

What for?

Thoughts circle during the day, cannot get out, cannot get anywhere. At night they're free. For several hours in the early morning everything comes clear. I don't want to miss that opportunity. I lie in wait; it keeps being given to me.

Do you believe you have special powers?

Not superpowers but I see very clearly at 3 a.m.

Do you hear voices or imagine presences?

What, you mean like burglars or extra-terrestrial beings? No, but I listen to Leonard Cohen's voice on my laptop at that time. There's a clarity then. Everything is very connected and very clear.

November 2016: Lithium

Four chairs in a row like a test, a bright light over the desk, all medical details displayed on the monitor; nothing on the walls, all windows closed, all radiators on; heat overpowering, the psychiatrist's voice monotonous and lulling.

> *You will start the medication; then there will be weekly blood-tests to check the toxin levels. Dangers include respiratory depression, seizures, coma. Common side-effects include weight gain, tremors in your hands dry mouth, increased thirst or urination, nausea, vomiting, loss of appetite, stomach pain, changes in your skin or hair, impotence, feeling uneasy.*

DIARY OF A BIPOLAR EXPLORER

Voice slowing down radiators humming nothing on the walls or floors white light flickering overhead radiators throbbing too hot in here voice continuous sleep coming please sleep coming...

> *Toxicity is lethal. Even a thimble of alcohol can cause renal failure. If you have any unusual symptoms, if you are off balance, check in immediately to A&E. Don't take any chances.*

No doors or windows in the walls. What do you mean please by off balance? A trembling membrane thickens on my brain sleep coming please sleep coming please sleep coming.

Do you want to use my body as a gauge for your toxins? Am I your measured toxicity?

Where's my mind? Is it stored in some place that's separate from me, flexing like an eye in pain?

Stuff your leaflet stuff your weekly blood-tests stuff your monitoring stuff your weight gain stuff your A&E stuff your seizures stuff your coma stuff your impending renal failure.

Get me out of here I'll take a walk home in the rain.

CHAPTER FIVE: RETIREMENT AND BREAKDOWN

December 2016: A true friend

Where would I be in all this without Sandie? She's always there at the end of the telephone or ready to respond by e-mail. She listens to me, offers wise advice, reads everything I write and gives me feedback on it. We meet for lunch, for coffee; we go for walks. She questions my assumptions, unsettles my point of view, and above all makes me laugh. I don't deserve so stalwart and good a friend.

December 2016: Sleep

"Hello darkness, my old friend..." Sleep is indeed "the main thing" as the psychiatrist said in one of my consultations – and as I found to my cost in the hospital ward in Leeds in 2002. Insomnia night after night can gradually produce hypomania; extreme sleep-deprivation is a well-known torture and can induce psychosis. Every doctor and fellow bipolar sufferer I've ever talked to has confirmed that regular sleep is the key to managing mood-swings. However, while enjoying "elevated mood", as I am at the moment, the very last thing I want to be told is that I need more sleep. Doing without it opens up a number of new opportunities for the bipolar patient. There are more hours in the day for creative activity. At intervals there's a very sharp sense of clarity; and there's an increased sense of potential, of being able to accomplish more by being wide awake for longer.

I'm waking very early every morning. I've decided to get up every time this happens and write down my thoughts without censoring them, as a stream of consciousness. I will call this "automatic writing" even though technically it's not the same as the supernaturally inspired/explained writing of WB Yeats and Georgie Hyde-Lees. My psychiatrist would be against my doing this; I should be sleeping. But the medication I've been put on makes me restless, so I can't help being awake and I want to use my time well. Here's what I wrote earlier this morning. I'll keep writing into my diary if the pattern of sleeplessness continues:

> *I went to bed early and slept till one, waking to know myself alone, even here among my family. Half a poem lay forming in the darkness until I slept again, waking briefly at two. At this hour the comparing power of the mind is gone, all proportion lost in dazzling sharpness. I woke again at three, no Syrian refugee, but homeless among sleeping Oxford houses.*

CHAPTER FIVE: RETIREMENT AND BREAKDOWN

When I tracked my own home down I found it hidden,
almost forgotten, along a pathway of autumnal lavenders.
I could see inside; my daughter was preparing a meal for
two, and my husband was typing. I was the monster in
Frankenstein, *the ghost in* The Sixth Sense *for ever*
shut outside. I learned to cook by watching through the
window, miming. By lip-reading I could listen to my
daughter calling her dad to supper.

If I had stayed awake, if I had only stayed awake
and written my next thoughts down, I would not then
have known (at six, waking restless and forlorn) the
sense of something stolen or forsaken. I had missed my
nightly tryst with darkness; my sharpest thoughts were
left un-tasted. Oh Sleep! You have so much to answer for.
Look at these three long hours you've wasted.

December 2016: Automatic writing

Darkness throughout the house as I tiptoe along the landing
to my study, making sure not to wake the others. I like the early
morning silence, with no-one about except our anxious cat.
It's curious how, at this hour and having only just awoken, my
unconscious seems to draw on the poetry I've been reading
or that I know very well. I just let the pen move across the
paper and out comes a load of writing that has recognisable

161

poetic metre (and sometimes even rhyme) even though it's just a flow of words. Here's a small excerpt from today's:

> *I missed my tryst with darkness once again and woke at dawn, dismayed to find that three branching threads in which I'd gathered dreams were lost, and scattered now to the four winds. While sleeping I had traced these branching threads back to a single source, where thoughts had moved smooth and sedate as Yeats's swans, drifting apart in dawn's first probing light. Oh Sleep, you have ravelled thoughts together and have left upon my sleeve the traces of your flight. A sonnet could have formed last night – instead of which, these blank verse wandering lines which move because they must despite my mind that interrupts and questions what I think. I sit and write; I use for the first time in many years this fountain-pen, this ink.*

December 2016: The bailiff

Sometimes when I wake in the early hours and start writing there seems to be a battle between my body and my thoughts, with sleep trying to overcome me. I've begun to see sleep as the enemy of creativity:

I'm despised in the workplace. The doctor is fanatical, foretelling doom. My daughter breathes my despair. My husband works overtime on my receipts, repayments, taxes. And all this while the wall is growing stronger, not brick by brick but day by day. If it could be touched it would be my own. It grows around me, rarely seen but always known.

Sleep, you're a bailiff who has driven me into a corner. I can feel my eyes closing as I write. You're more powerful for being withheld from sight. If this were an allegory of stigma alone I could undo you, brick by brick, but it's also a fable of betrayal by sleep, and of the way that sleep is used by doctors to wage war on madness.

Wakefulness is a fiery gift which can un-build all walls. Look! How easily the wall between the public and the private is torn down.

January 2017: Reams

We're at our cottage in Cornwall; it's icy cold in the early hours, even when the fire has succeeded in keeping going. At first the change of scenery and the very pure air seemed to settle me, so I slept well. Now I'm waking through the night, just as I did at home. The silence is thicker here as I get up to write. I need a hot water bottle beside me as I sit scribbling:

I wake each day at 3.00, believing I've written reams on reams of thoughts; that all they need now is to be moved from my writing-pad to my PC and from there to the Forum. I long for completion. In the first five minutes as I lie in bed I feel sure, quite sure, I'll find them. As I get up I'm still convinced they're here. Making tea I watch the pendulum swing to and fro while silence thickens in the dark outside and wonder if all writing is a dream. As I settle to the clock's loud tick I begin to be certain that yesterday is on repeat; that there's a loop in history and this is Groundhog Day. All I've so far written is being deleted then re-written, but not by me. My words are no longer mine: who is making away with them? Is this the meaning of interpretation? By the time I open my PC, I've come to full awareness, and I don't search for what will not be there. The dawn will soon have come. I know full well by now that as before I'll find my dream-script gone: scattered about by time to the four winds and on a foreign shore.

CHAPTER FIVE: RETIREMENT AND BREAKDOWN

January 2017: The consultation

Back in Oxford now, and trying to get back to regular pattern of sleep. I'm having some success. It's icy cold out in the streets and as I walk back from the Warneford my eyes stream with tears. I think of a man I saw yesterday in the city centre, curled up asleep in a doorway in full daylight among a pile of newspapers: two sleeping-bags not enough to keep him warm; his begging cup overturned because there was no one around when he was last awake.

I feel porous and vulnerable; but oh, how I like my new psychiatrist! She's gentle and wise; her face keeps breaking into a smile even when I'm not trying to be funny. If I ask her a basic question she doesn't give a basic answer, but a whole tutorial – pitching the level high, using technical vocabulary. She's clever and kind, she understands a mood disorder as if from inside. When she talks of receptors it's as if she knows them and she said the phrase "partial agonist" with pride. (I asked her to write it down for me, so I could turn it into poetry.) I've seen her three times and already I feel she knows me. When I refused the lithium she didn't try to persuade. When I told her that I *enjoy* going without sleep, she seemed to sympathise. She wants me to sleep but doesn't want to make me. How I fear for my new psychiatrist! She's so patient and generous with her time. How come she has a whole hour to go through all this with me? She's a high-level researcher; how will she survive? Great clinicians are extremely rare, I'm told. She's worth her weight in goodness, not in gold.

January 2017: Storytelling

I wrote the following story a few weeks before outing my Bipolar Disorder on the Hall Writers' Forum. Now, looking back, it reads as if it's about the history of my illness, though I had no consciousness of its being so at the time. The way it emerged, day after day, had a strange kind of inevitability, as if it had been waiting for years to be written. I still don't understand the cruelty that was uncovered in myself in the course of writing this. All I know is that I can be cruel. Violence seems to be a recurring theme in this diary.

Three pigeons in a box

During the day they made a placid sound (sometimes asleep) inside the box between the window and my bed – their soft "coos" subdued, their wings folded. I often thought, as I listened to the warm contentment in their

166

day-time pulse, of incubation. At night the quiet cooing stopped. When it was my turn to sleep they began their fluttering, their agitated scratching and pecking below the padlocked lid, while I lay watching the box in the dark as it shook and trembled. I knew them for what they were by the fact that they never ate, or shat; and I resented them only a little. Over the years I began to fear that if I let them out they might by then have lost their silvery sheen. Better to shelter them than to see their plumage.

Inside the box it was warm and dark, light creeping through the cracks during the daytime. They had room enough to move about, each with a favourite corner. They took comfort in each other's bodies. With no memory of trees, of sky, of grass, they knew only my shufflings outside the box, the gradations of light as I opened or closed the curtains. They felt attuned to my steady rhythms. When the long strange silence began each night, pitch-blackness closing in like prison, they took turns watching. They needed to get out. It was only a matter of time before they'd wear the walls down with the beating of their wings.

One spring when the warmer weather came the cooing inside the box by day became louder, more continuous, and interspersed with busy sounds of re-

furbishing. I concluded they must be nesting. At night they were quieter and I sensed that they were watching. This break in their settled joint routine was mildly disconcerting so I dragged the box through from the bedroom to the box-room, where there was almost total darkness. As I moved I could sense them going still. I could feel the weight of their bodies. After that I slept more easily at night and although I missed the steady throb of their daytime cooing I checked the padlock and kept the door firmly locked, feeling in need of clearer boundaries. The days passed languorously, I re-discovered gardening.

They had known darkness before and they had known silence – but never this profound. In the box, inside the box room, all they could hear was themselves. They remained for a long time unaccountably still. But as the days passed they grew accustomed to cooing nervously in turns and to sleeping in shifts, listening for the soft footfall of spiders. Weeks passed. They eyed each other with wary over-familiarity. Never till now had they thought of mating. Never till now had they felt hunger. They watched, they waited.

I spent the long summer months mostly outside, tending the garden and drawing birds – a woodpecker, robins and sparrows, the occasional jay. I liked to hang these on my walls. They were intricate and consoling; they paid close attention to eyes and claws. During the day-time I easily forgot the box hidden in the box-room. But when I lay between sleep and waking I could sometimes hear a plaintive, low, coo-cooing sound, the rhythmic peck of beak on wood, the muffled beat of wings along the corridor. (A black cat now slept between my bed and the window, where the box had been. Its insolent indifference to me and to the sounds that worried me was a kind of insurance. If the birds were real, would he not be scratching hungrily, persistently, at the box-room door?)

As the days shortened, dust gathering inside the box-room, filmy cobwebs hung between the cornice and the door-frame. But inside the darkness, inside the silence, the long slow waiting finally stopped. Was it the gradual attrition of time, or the frustrated flapping of wings, or the combined power of three hungry beaks, that had worn away the joins? Their claws were enough, now, to prise open the box. One by one, blinking and astonished, they tiptoed out into their capacious prison. There was no wild beating of wings; no jubilation; but shyly, cautiously, two of them began a courtship dance...

169

I moved downstairs to be away from the noises. My sitting room became my bedroom. As time passed I often forgot the difference between night and day, sleeping through the boundaries. I'd lie in bed, whiling away the hours, watching the garden through the window. I wasn't drawing anymore and I had no visitors. I'd carefully selected three or four songs I liked, which I played over and over. I was conserving energy, frugally making a shortlist of memories I felt were necessary, that would serve me the rest of my life-time. I collected leaves from the garden and pressed them. I had sheaves of these, ranged on my bookshelves. Their dried life pleased me. Finding everything I needed on the ground floor I had no occasion to make the journey upstairs. Gradually the noises faded.

In the box room there was an adequate supply of spiders. Occasionally a mouse, happening along by chance, provided food and entertainment. Mating came naturally: two birds paired for life, the other watched enviously. The first egg hatched well, providing food for all three; after that the cycle of reproduction and digestion was steady, with enough chicks to ensure survival. Half were instant food, the rest lived to breed. Sometimes fights broke out, especially among the original three over petty details, such as the pecking order. There were no disputes over territory. A system evolved for rotational nesting inside a broken guitar.

Was it months or years since I'd vacated the upstairs bedroom, to avoid the reminders? By now I'd lost all sense of time: each day passed so quietly that I'd found a kind of peace. What was it, then, that awoke me suddenly one morning? The smell came first and then the flapping. It was there continuously, close to my brain – as if a moth, trapped in my ear, were beating its helpless wings. The more it rustled, the stronger came the scent, sweet and sickly. I found a word for the sound, which haunted me all morning: "sussuration". Knowing that sooner or later I must go upstairs, I longed to have the cat with me for the journey.

On the landing I paused. There was no sound inside the box-room. And yet my mind, like a room, was full of low cooings, soft downy flutterings, so that even before opening the door I sensed with a sudden flash of foreknowledge what I would find. I stood on the threshold, braced and steadied for the transfiguration. Inside, on every surface, countless pigeons perched, preening their blue-grey plumage, which shone in the semi-darkness like dusky silver. The room rocked gently to the motion of their rustling wings, to the steady thrum of their incessant cooing. Beside the broken box lay a mound of bones, the chewed remains of pigeon carcasses; and strewn all round among the droppings, layer upon layer of grey feathers, heads with staring eyes, and gristly claws.

I tiptoed gently in, no longer trembling but strangely calm, and opened the skylight. A wintry sun flooded the cobwebbed room. The cat arrived just in time to see me turning for one last look as I closed and locked the door.

Chapter Six:
Re-visitings

Deepest winter. In our frozen road the blue pipes lie exposed like giant arteries. Two men excavate, stamping along the edge of a deep open wound. Noise-maddened, small birds huddle or shiver, pecking hard at the feeder…

In the aftermath of outing my illness on the Forum, I'm drawn to re-visiting my patterns of behaviour across the years since diagnosis. Some of these reassessments are coming in the form of poems. Poetry helps me to analyse and distil my emotions: the mental energy I expend on this is more constructive than simply going over and over the feelings without articulating them. The villanelle is a form in which obsessional thought-patterns can be expressed through insistent circling refrains. Posting this poem on the Hall Writers' Forum has been, in a strange way, exhilarating: it's a relief to be able to look back on my life and write openly about abnormal behaviour:

Diary of a Bipolar Explorer

The addict's debt

I managed for ten years without, and yet
I looked for novel ways to keep me sane.
My need continued; still I ran up debt.

Wine was forgetfulness, easy to get –
a draught the readiest thing to drain.
I managed for ten years without, and yet

when I stopped drinking, I was newly set
on finding ways to numb a hidden pain.
My need continued. Still I ran up debt.

Now I was thin and elegant, I let
myself indulge in clothes and shoes again –
I'd managed for ten years without, and yet

they soon appealed. No one I've ever met
could spend so lavishly on being vain!
My need continued, still I ran up debt.

When each enthusiasm "ended", I would bet
my life that I was free of its dark bane.
I'd manage, now, ten years without! And yet

a new craze always surfaced: keeping fit,
books, paintings, CDs – nothing I'd disdain:
my need continued, still I ran up debt.

CHAPTER SIX: RE-VISITINGS

What is this hunger to consume, this threat
that spills itself and spreads like a dark stain?
I've managed for ten years without! And yet

I know full well the cycle will repeat
over and over − I'll not break the chain.
My need continues. Still I run up debt.

And now this Forum has become my dearest pet,
my best addiction - No, I can't refrain!
I manage for ten hours without - and yet
my need continues. Still I run up debt.

January 2017: Flouting the doctors

Crocuses in full bloom under denuded apple trees; bees by the score, sipping the nectar in sunshine... this early spring is welcome, even if deceptive. I find myself in tune with the garden, attentive to the changes there as if they were bound up with my moods.

Currently the last thing I want is medication. I'd prefer to be entirely myself with the ups and downs than wandering around in a dazed and confused state produced by pills. Disobeying doctors' orders and neglecting medication are quite common faults among those who have Bipolar Disorder because of the long-term nature of the condition, which makes us resent being tied to a regime. There's also some evidence that the most effective medication interferes with creativity. Being very active is sometimes a sign that hypomania is arriving. There's always a choice to be made between being balanced through medicine and being riskily creative. I've written this in imitation of Emily Dickinson, who may well have suffered from BD.

The self now seeing

They hide behind their shiny screens
to muse, and gloze, and pry –
a little clan of medicine men
whose hospital's hard by.

I see them in my nightmares
in suits and serried rows.
They trap me with their lures and snares –
until the black mood goes.

My stock of little poison-pills
tucked in their plastic sheet
and covered in thin metal foil –
it tempts me, "Come and eat!"

I'm stupefied by medicine –
my numbed brain put on hold.
My limbs are like a mannequin's –
I wander, dull and cold.

Five months go past; there is a wall
that grows with time more wide.
till February comes – and still
no warmth can get inside.

But now the poison-pills are done –
I'll have no more of them.
The serried rows of suits are gone –
Dismissed, upon a whim.

Prescribe me nothing. I am free
to flout this world of men –
and spring is here to welcome me
back to my blues again.

January 2017: Writing and illness

I find it harder to write about my illness in relation to other people than to immerse myself in the symptoms and explore them from the inside. This condition is so egocentric and isolating. Imagining how others see us when we're ill is tricky and insight can sometimes be lost. This next poem is written in response to advice from a Forum friend to write about my marriage – the way it has been affected by the illness and how it survives. I've invented the form I use here (an adaptation of the kyrielle). Before writing the poem I had a conversation with Martin, who observes my mood-swings carefully and takes care of me very well.

Ringing the changes

I asked him why he stays with me
when I withdraw from company,
and all is difficult and strange.
He smiled and said "Such things must be.
I married you; you married me.
I love you and that doesn't change".

I asked him why he doesn't go
out where the warm winds softly blow
to find new life and widely range.
He smiled and said, "You surely know
even when you are really low
I love you and that doesn't change."

I asked him would he take the vow
if he knew then what he knows now –
that I am sick, and often strange.
He smiled and said "We cannot know.
I see your faults now. Even so
I love you and that doesn't change."

I told him what I always knew:
without his help, what would I do?
All full-time care's beyond my range.
He laughed and said "That's very true.
I'm glad, then, to look after you.
I love you and that doesn't change."

The next poem is written in the sestina form, which has no rhymes; the poem is held into unity by a very strict rotating pattern of end-words in each line. I've turned to the sestina here because I want to suggest patterns of repetition within the marriage that are determined by my illness. The discipline of writing in this strict rhyme-less form has helped to give a shape to inchoate feelings.

Diary of a Bipolar Explorer

A lunchtime conversation

"I married you, you married me; we are together
And we have a daughter", he said, as we lunched
on soup and ciabatta in the cold. "I won't lie.
I don't like your forum", he said, "but I like you
and that doesn't change, even when you're sick.
When you come through, there's a bit of balance."

"You may find it difficult to maintain balance
and that's not the sickness' fault altogether –
there is more to your writing than being sick…"
He paused mid-sentence as we sat at lunch,
talking of our marriage and the future. "You
are never beyond my hope; but I won't lie –

It would be wrong, talking of these things, to lie.
I love you and that doesn't change, but I need you
to work harder on staying sane, on keeping balance.
Please make more effort." His words, as we sat together,
were chilling. There was a stillness as we lunched,
talking of what he feels and does when I am sick.

It's true, I am not always or altogether sick;
and as we talk of this again we mustn't lie.

CHAPTER SIX: RE-VISITINGS

We felt the need, talking today as we lunched
to create a new understanding, a new balance
which came out of our being so long together.
"I want to see much more", he explained "of you" –

"not your forum, not your poetry, but you,
and it's only through control, when you're sick,
that we can have a proper life together."
He talked seriously and he did not lie;
his face was gentle and we found our balance
as we sat facing each other and calmly lunched.

Did something new happen today as we lunched?
Does this betoken something different? "Will you
remind me that I've felt this sense of balance
when I'm next in danger of being really sick?
I want a panacea that does not lie,
I want a way of staying well together."

To remain addicted to the forum is to stay sick;
it is to deceive you. It is, after this lunch, to lie.
That is no way of being balanced together.

February 2017: Writing and taboo

Something has triggered an obsession with the past. I'm going over and over the events of that morning in Leeds when I was sectioned for psychosis. The Forum is still my main outlet and this is how I express my feelings there:

> *What would have happened if, instead of calling an ambulance, my mother had instead let me have a quiet sleep in her flat in Chapel Allerton? Then I would not have had to go through the indignity of being carted off in an ambulance like a maniac, subjected to the sign "DOMESTIC WASTE ONLY" and watched throughout my incarceration in mental hospital by an eye in the door. Is this whole illness of mine made worse by my own and others' terror of insanity? Would it in fact have been a whole lot better for me and my family if this diagnosis had not been made? We're all human; acute distress can cause strange behaviour -- and sleep can be a great tonic, even in some cases a healer.*

The positive outcome of self-analysis and Forum discussion is more openness with my mum and sisters. Revisiting trauma in conversation with them spells the beginning of the end for a family taboo.

CHAPTER SIX: RE-VISITINGS

A taboo is a prohibition on thoughts, on words, on actions: a collective means of dealing with our deepest fears by classifying them as unmentionable. How do we know a taboo when we see it? If a topic comes up in conversation and an embarrassed unease shows in body language. If someone swallows hard, and a deep silence follows. If they delay in answering, or prevaricate. If they flannel, or fail to respond, or hesitate to come to the rescue. And so we replace our transgressions with Bad Faith and its familiar toxins: *"Cover it up, cover it up please, miss. No one is ready yet to talk about this."* Oh, to breathe freely, to feel and know there's no censorship, no embargo! No more pussy-footing round the dark and dangerous pit that opens up when we allude to *it*.

What exactly happened that day in Leeds when I was sectioned? How does everyone in the family feel about it? The topic has always been an elephant in the room, at least when I've been present. Piecing things together now, I understand that there has been discussion of it amongst some family members; but so far as I myself have been concerned, the subject has been one on which people have fallen silent — out of embarrassment perhaps, but it has *felt* as though the psychosis is a disgrace, a source of collective shame. It's not until now, in 2017, that it has

183

become possible to share in detail what happened. How strange to find this topic up for family discussion at last! As we enter this phase of openness, whose words are any of us to trust? There were four of us involved: there are now four women's narratives.

February 2017: Revisiting the Showdown

The psychosis was fifteen years ago, yet the emotions connected with it feel as fresh as yesterday and I live in double time, a kind of nightmare. Each of the poems below has emerged out of conversation with a member of my family about that day in Leeds. The poems are presented in the order of composition. They trace an evolving response on my part to family conflicts. The creative process was set in motion by my desire to have everything out in the open. But how vulnerable I am to other people's narratives, given that there is a part of what happened that I can never retrieve! It was a revelation to discover that one of my sisters, Gill, was not there at the flat in Chapel Allerton when the police and ambulance were called to take me away. She had stayed behind at St James's hospital (despite acute pain in her eyes at this time) to keep a vigil at our dad's bedside. This is a poem for Gill, to thank her for not being part of the process that led to my being sectioned:

The threshold

Three steps from the driveway to the hall.
Only a threshold to cross into a home,
and only a door between.

I am a blank, I am forgotten; my actions
are reconstructed from Chinese whispers,
I have no hold on what they are, or mean.

Three steps into the hallway from the drive
and only the door between myself and sleep,
which will rescue me from madness.

Was I silent, or did I scream? Did my sister really
hold me down, to restrain my violence?
I have no memory of this, only reconstructions.

Once across the threshold, I would have been
asleep, dead to the world in a cosy bed
instead of dumped like rubbish in a looney bin.

Can I picture the whole scene differently
now I know you were not there? Can I
imagine you, alone for hours on the ward –

your eyes sore and your heart in pain?
Will this help me, so that I walk up the steps
to find that other person I might have been

waiting for me, re-born at the other side –
wide awake now, refreshed after long sleep,
and ready to face the day?

I've been over and over that morning.
The threshold can never be made clean.
But now for the first time I find you

outside the blank, in the ward with dad –
unknowing, intensely loved, and real.
I need no longer stay away.

To realise that Gill was not implicated in my removal and subsequent sectioning has been a huge relief to me. However, in talking to her I've become aware that she went through her own traumas that night. I've used a favourite form, the villanelle, to capture the obsessive circling of her thoughts as she sat in the hospital ward with dad.

Gill's vigil

Her eyes were sore, and her heart was broken.
Now that he had her with him at his side
she thought only of the last time they had spoken.

The turbulence had ended, but was re-awoken
with no one there in whom she could confide.
Her eyes were sore, and her heart was broken.

Chapter Six: Re-visitings

What would they both do, should he awaken
and find her there, with no one else beside?
She thought only of the last time they had spoken –

his anger; her fear of all that was left open
unfolding there for ever while he died.
Her eyes were sore, and her heart was broken

by all her recent wounds, which made her weaken:
she couldn't find forgiveness, though she tried.
She thought only of the last time they had spoken.

Nursing her ache, discounting every token
of love for fear that it was empty or it lied,
her eyes were sore, and her heart was broken.
She thought only of the last time they had spoken.

The next two sestinas are to be read as a pair; they narrate the perspectives of my mother and my sister Kate respectively. Listening to their accounts, an incompatibility in their memories has emerged – perhaps due to the amount of time that has elapsed since the events took place? I'm not clear yet if this pair of poems is evidence of my unrelenting grudge about that never to be forgotten day in Leeds or a sign that I'm beginning to move beyond the traumatic memory. Only time will tell.

DIARY OF A BIPOLAR EXPLORER

The spectacle

I jibbed at the thought of being a spectacle.
Going over it all in my mind yet again,
I asked her, was I quiet or was I screaming?
Did she call the ambulance or the police from here?
I needed to sleep – I wasn't a maniac.
Why hadn't she allowed me to come inside?

"You refused to budge, you refused to go inside.
All eyes at the windows watched the spectacle
of you gripping me with your iron clutch like a maniac.
You yelled You're the only one again and again.
Kate dialled 999: We have an hysteric here.
You had me in your iron clutch; you were screaming.

When the police-car came, you were still screaming;
an ambulance man coaxed you briefly inside.
Eyes watched the whole thing unfolding here
as if it were a drama, or a spectacle –
everyone woken by sirens wailing again and again;
and you inside now, talking like a maniac.

When they carried you away, you were still a maniac
but quieter now, you were no longer screaming;

Chapter Six: Re-visitings

I said I don't know what to do *again and again,*
sitting shocked and still on my own inside,
lost for a long time to myself, outside the spectacle –
as if I'd had a stroke, part of me no longer here."

I imagine her sitting stunned, all alone in there
having just seen her daughter like a maniac
and I'm no longer haunted by the spectacle
of hugging her with my massive hug and screaming.
I feel only her lonely shock as she sits inside,
going over the scene in her mind all over again.

What was she going to do, she asked again;
What would this mean, where would we all go from here?
When we were on the ward, all of us inside,
would dad have heard my screaming like a maniac?
Was he woken, was he disturbed by my screaming?
Did he know, was he aware of the spectacle?

This time, as I re-imagine the spectacle,
I see the maniac again– no longer screaming
at the forbidden threshold, but there with mum, inside.

Diary of a Bipolar Explorer

Kate's testimony

Was I screaming when we left the hospital?
Was I still screaming loudly outside the flat?
Was it Kate who dialled 999? Was there violence?
Did she call the police because she was frightened?
Did she come with me in the ambulance?
These were the details I asked her to reveal.

And as we talked, to see what she could reveal,
we made discoveries: "No screaming in hospital,
only while we waited for the ambulance;
only while I held you down, using force outside the flat."
Yes. I'd been strange: she'd been very frightened –
enough to pull me down by my hair. Such violence.

I'd hugged mum so hard she must use violence.
"We have an hysteric here": she could now reveal
mum had used those words, not she. "We were frightened.
Mum hadn't known anything was wrong in hospital,
only when you arrived back, upset, at the flat
and she saw the need for police and an ambulance."

When the men had arrived in the ambulance
it was then I was screaming – at Kate's violence.
I had already been with her and mum inside the flat
(yes, this she could absolutely reveal.)
I'd been agitated since leaving hospital,
talking in sudden jerks; I'd made her frightened.

190

CHAPTER SIX: RE-VISITINGS

"You were hugging mum so tight – she was so frightened
that I had to hold you down and call the ambulance
to take you away and put you into hospital..."
No, she wouldn't say that what she'd done was violence.
There were a number of things she could reveal:
I'd paced and talked about Strange Meeting *while in the flat.*

Nothing could contain my agitation in the flat.
They had both been so extremely frightened.
This she could herself one hundred per cent reveal:
I'd screamed only while they waited for the ambulance.
She had been forced to use such violence
To ensure that I was taken away to hospital.

She came, frightened, with the men to hospital.
Her hand shook when she signed the form. Such violence.
Had she been right, at the flat, to call the ambulance?

If the two people who were most awake that morning can't
agree on what happened, how can we as a family process and
come to terms with it? The only thing that seems completely
clear from conversations is this: both mum and Kate believe
that the team on the ward where dad lay dying should have
taken more responsibility for my state of mind and called
a psychiatrist to care for me. I can see their point of view,
but is this a disowning of their own responsibility as family
members? Wasn't this a *domestic* crisis? Why should there be

any expectation that my distress could be handled by staff on a busy ward looking after the patients in their care? For me the experience of being sectioned was shattering and the actions taken by my mother and by Kate are still hard to accept. But each member of the family has been affected by the direct and indirect repercussions of my illness, so this perhaps influences the opinions of all parties.

In the aftermath of these discussions and revelations we're collectively dismayed to find that our stories won't cohere. Each of us has an emotional investment in our own point of view. As we try hard to rescue the underlying facts of what happened, the tug of our individual perspectives interferes with our capacity to see the other sides. We pull in different directions, trying to claim or publicly disown a sad and meagre advantage. Which are the key words here as I begin to imagine a book in print – and is this a family story? Am I one person asking permission to speak for all of us in a master narrative that we must all confirm? Or am I *myself* alone, damaged and fighting my corner in a superseded contest? If our memories were a palimpsest there might be hope of an ultimate moment of recovery – but all the lines are jumbled, criss-crossed, spiralling. Even as I commit to one version it's already shadowy or lost: compelled and revised by what seems valid in another. History is like this. There's no truth; only the various stories, tugging and tugging at the narrator's conscience: claim and counter-claim struggling for recognition.

How can there be such a thing as reconciliation within this protracted process? We watch and wait; the emails fly backward, forward – no one exactly losing their cool; no one entirely baring her soul. All are shocked and wary; one seems almost completely withdrawn. It may be wrong to hope for some kind of catharsis. We may have reached a kind of impasse in interpretation and communication which can never be fully overcome.

Minute by Minute

Thoughts, they say, are free – like
air, like rain-water, like common land.
Obsessions, though, are like the grains
of sand in an hourglass: trapped,
and moving in one direction
only, not through volition but
by force of gravity. A pucker,
a dimple in the sand's surface
widens to a hollow, tapers
to a thread, tugged steadily
from below. Minute by
minute you watch
its slow trickle,
mesmerized
by the
in-
evitable
momentum,
the obvious drift.
And then just as it's
finished, just as the cone
above is replaced in a sudd-
en rush, and almost identically
by the cone beneath, you turn
the whole thing over, and watch
it happen again. Self-renewing
and self - depleting, this sand
goes nowhere, soundlessly:
gaining nothing and losing nothing,
like an obsession, e n d l e s s l y.

Chapter Seven:
Adjustment

Why should I let the toad "retirement" squat on my life? Just because my career has ended does this make me a superannuated woman? I still wake up each morning ready to get to work; I still want to undertake writing projects and earn rewards; I still look for the self-respect that comes from labour. And yes, I still hanker for the tiredness that ends each day. If you tell me that writing doesn't count as work, if you tell me that I'm just indulging myself at my leisure, I don't know how to answer you, or make your prejudice go away. You may be right. But have a care how you talk about us oldies. We're still here; we'll be knocking around for a good while yet. We're not just gardening, cooking, watching day-time TV and having lunch with friends. We still have things to plan, things to do, things to imagine and accomplish, things to write and say.

Diary of a Bipolar Explorer

March 2017: Writing

March is an ambiguous month; I can readily enter into its mood-swings. But gradually, day by day, I'm reaching some kind of internal stability with the help of medication, writing and the weather…

Behind the roadworks
a rich almond tree spreads wide
its laden branches.

The fragile blossoms
quietly promise more than
this uncertain spring.

I'm more and more reclusive. I find that I must write poetry regularly to keep sane. If I go a day without giving shape to my thoughts and moods I lose my sense of purpose – and then there's nothing to do but pace around the house. I seem unable to read for more than fifteen minutes at a time. Restlessness used to find an outlet in teaching. Now, in retirement, writing is the best anchor I can find. Sometimes all I need to do to balance my mood is write a single haiku about life in the garden. A haiku is the most distilled form there is: concentrating on it is a form of mindfulness. By linking my haikus together in a sequence

Chapter Seven: Adjustment

I can produce something like a garden diary in which my own moods are clearly traceable.

Far away from here
in the mind's spacious garden
stock-doves are mating.

Rose-stems arch and fan,
sending out their leaflets like
urgent messages.

Sun warms the pear-tree,
and the corms of irises
put up their green flags.

I'm also steadied by a couple of other creative projects. One is a collection of poems and songs about Bob Dylan written by members of the Hall Writers' Forum: I'm editing these, and will be publishing them at my own expense as a pamphlet. The second is less collaborative. I'm putting together a series of poems about landscape painters in the nineteenth century: Turner, Constable, Cotman, Palmer, Cozens and Towne. So far I have forty-five poems. Each focuses on a single painting, interpreting its creative principles. In writing, I become completely absorbed in these paintings, almost as if I'm their creator.

Diary of a Bipolar Explorer

I find tranquillity in observation and interpretation. I'm taken entirely out of myself in writing. Is it significant that this feeling of being more settled comes with thinking about *painting*? I used to be a passably good watercolourist; perhaps my poems are telling me to open up my sketchbooks and paint-boxes once again. There are times when writers need to get beyond words.

April 2017: My last lecture

I'm back from an academic conference in Cardiff and depleted after an exhausting week. I always find the build-up to academic conferences tricky, even when I'm due to give a lecture on a topic well within my expertise. This one, a plenary, involved talking about Edward Thomas and Wordsworth. It took me away from home for four nights, making me restless and unhappy. I was so stressed on the day I had to travel that I got to the station an hour before I needed to, having misinterpreted the train schedule. Later I sat on the train reading terrible predictions in the news of World War III. I've been chewing a lot of nicorettes lately, trying to get over my sudden addiction to smoking which set in last November. While travelling I got through more of these than was good for me and arrived at my hotel somewhat over-stimulated.

Chapter Seven: Adjustment

Cardiff is a city of gulls. From the hotel window I watched them wheeling about, calling among the roof-tops. With nothing better to do it was freedom enough to see them flying or strutting on the high ledges as they preened themselves in the sun. If it hadn't been for the scent of sea from the bay their companionable cries would have been drowned out by other sensations. But they were so close, their wings flapping just outside my top-floor window, that they haunted my thoughts like a waking dream. Beneath the ledge a wire mesh stretched from the hotel to the building opposite, stopping the birds from flying too near. But a careless gap, wide enough to serve as a trap, ran the full length of the street. As darkness fell, my room filled with fear. I imagined the muffled flap of a gull caught under the net alone. In my sleep I heard it struggling, beating its helpless wings in the tunnel, its wild cries stifled in the windless city night like an imprisoned soul. How thin the partition is between humans and birds! Captured in our web they have no place to hide. (If you're petrified by wings, then build a cage and put *yourself* inside. The air's not ours to portion and patrol.)

There were a few people at the conference I knew and more I'm glad to have got to know; but even so I felt anxious while I was there. I've never been so nervous about a public performance, except perhaps when I gave my first ever lecture at the age of 23 in front of Seamus Heaney. So despite the fact that this recent lecture went well I've resolved never to do one again. There's no need to subject myself to nerve-wracking tension now I'm retired. I can attend conferences without giving lectures; I can continue to publish academic work without being on the conference circuit. This resolution will help me manage the ongoing problems of the mood disorder as I grow older. (I'm happy to go on giving poetry readings when the opportunity arises, as I did this time in Cardiff. Nerves are much less of a problem when I'm reading my poems, for some reason that I don't fully understand.)

Breaking news! I "outed" my bipolarity at my lecture. Or rather, I asked the conference organiser who introduced me to let it be known that I'm writing about it in this book. I'm still not sure what led me to do this. Perhaps it was because I knew that it would be my last lecture and wanted in some way to explain myself to the audience. Perhaps it was just a joining up of dots to make my story complete in my own mind. I'm glad to have taken the step and I was proud to be thanked by members of the audience for being open. One of these was Gwyneth Lewis, whose book *Sunbathing in the Rain* is the best account of depression I know: it has proved something of a life-saver to me on a number of occasions. It was great to meet her and thank her for writing it.

May 2017: Discharge

I've been discharged from the outpatient clinic at the Warneford. My GP will supervise longer term care. As so often happens after an episode of hypomania I'm in a period of depression. This is likely to last for a while, as I know from experience.

The Dylan pamphlet has been published, so I have no immediate writing projects. I'm feeling discouraged by the process of trying to line up a publisher for my sonnets about the Wordsworths: the state of poetry in this country is worrying. I'm shocked and demoralised by the news that my poetry publisher has closed its poetry list, which will mean that I don't have a home for my poetry in future. (I heard this news in January but it has taken a long while for its implications to sink in.)

Medication is helping me to feel steady. The psychiatrist put me on an anti-psychotic drug as well as anti-depressants and this combination seems to work, but at the cost of my creativity. I'm currently unable to write, although concentration on reading is possible. Addictions are well under control; I sometimes go swimming. Reduced activity on the Forum is probably a good thing. As a consequence I've read seven Iris Murdoch novels in succession. I also notice that I'm taking more interest in the news and my family. I'm not filling in any of the mood graphs. I feel lost if I try to describe where I am on them.

June 2017: Offcomers

What does "home" signify? What is it to feel a sense of belonging? In retirement we have much more time at our cottage in Cornwall than we ever did before. The air is pure here in Veryan, and when we get out to the beach or the cliffs I feel invigorated by the sight and smell and sound of the sea. I love the gulls calling from roof-tops in the morning, the noisy rooks in the beech-trees by the pub at supper time. I love the tiny harbour at Portloe with its fishing boats and crab creels; I love walking with my shoes and socks off in the shallows at Carne and Pendower. Some of the local footpaths are becoming so familiar that I could find my way along them in the dark…But this to-ing and fro-ing between Oxford and Cornwall comes at a cost. My mood-swings are exacerbated by travel and sleep is disturbed for a few nights after the long drive. It feels like jet-lag: until I've been in one or other place for at least

Chapter Seven: Adjustment

a week I don't feel settled. Oxford seems less of a home because we spend less time there; and in Veryan I can't get rid of the pervasive feeling of being an outsider looking in.

This place is being taken over by offcomers ("blow-ins" as they're known in Ireland) – and we're among them. The luxury of being a second home-owner fills me with unease and guilt – not only because of the millions of homeless people in the world, but because of the havoc wrought on the local Cornish economy by gentrification. My guilty conscience will persist until we sell our Oxford house and make a permanent move to this village. But can I imagine doing that? The place could never truly be home; I could never uproot from the city I've lived in for over forty years.

Offcomers

You can tell who we are, even a long way off,
by our unlit windows. We have model
fishing-boats on prominent display,
with absurd collections of large shells.

Our walking-boots wait for us,
visible in our porches, together with
walking-sticks and torches. Our log-piles
are stacked away, tidy and neat, in sheds nearby.

DIARY OF A BIPOLAR EXPLORER

We are herded together at the wrong end
of the village – an offcomer colony,
speeding up and down the motorways
to our hidey-holes here on the Cornish coast.

We've bought nearly all the houses
in the most picturesque villages, where
the only locals run the pubs. In the winter
they are deserted. The chapels are ghosts.

We nod to the villagers, known as friendly folk.
We have mates among them, sometimes
join them for a drink. We pride ourselves
on being people the farmers will greet.

Always, this sense of being between
two places, reluctant bystanders in both.
The gulls circle overhead, querying, querying,
as we clean the cottage and pack our bags to leave.

"Freshly clicked" the Tesco's van announces,
pulling up outside our neighbour's house
while down in the village shop the dust collects
among un-bought vegetables and fruit.

Chapter Seven: Adjustment

June 2017: Politics

Austerity bites hard in this benighted country. Every day I read reports in the news of savage cuts to the NHS, with their disastrous consequences. It's particularly upsetting to learn of the appalling shortage of funding for treatment of physical and mental disabilities.

Despite the fact that the Tories win, the results of the General Election are uplifting. I'm inspired not just by the Labour Party's manifesto but by the strength of Jeremy Corbyn's leadership. He's a brilliant campaigner and it's wonderful to listen to his rousing speeches at rallies. It seems as if – for the first time in living memory – a politician might soon get into power who can be wholly trusted. I've re-joined the Labour Party after a long period away from it. I follow the news closely. I can imagine being active in the future, especially if (as seems likely) there's another election soon.

The fire in Grenfell Tower horrifies and obsesses me. I check hourly for updates and am losing sleep. Nightmare images from the media fill my brain. There's one incident in particular – that of a woman who threw her baby to safety from the ninth floor – that I can't get out of my head. There's no symbol more resonant than that of the ejection of an infant by its mother. I go over and over the moral and emotional issues. Was her action a sudden reflex? How did she overcome her more natural instinct, to stay with her child to the death? What was her process of reasoning? Her presence of mind (desperate as she was, and terrified by such horrific circumstances) is heart-rending; as is the evidence of the whole local community coming together to look after the victims of the fire. I have an email correspondence with a Forum friend about the moral and political perplexities. His clarity helps me to get critical purchase. I'm so grateful for this.

Safe landing

The mum who dropped her baby from the tower
still haunts my dreams and every waking hour.
I've heard it said that when she threw you down
you landed safe below in arms unknown.

I cannot for your sake imagine this:
what pain before the binding farewell kiss?
What anguish as you hurtled through the air
and did she see you landing safely there?

CHAPTER SEVEN: ADJUSTMENT

The upheld arms of one who gave his all
to save your fragile life after the fall
may well have been her cherished final sight
before she choked to death that ghastly night.

I hope, though, that she lived and found her way
out of the blaze into the wakening day
and that her baby in the shell-shocked queue
is held in her arms now. Let this be true.

The only comfort if she died is this:
she reasoned well before her good-bye kiss.
Better a single death (her own) than two;
no other life more dear to her than you.

I see her choking as the flames shoot high,
the black smoke rushing in. All round her lie
the charred remains of the un-numbered dead.
Is she among them? Nothing has been said.

The black tower looms against the London sky,
holding its secrets still as months go by.
Hers is one story. There are many more
who lost their lives that night for being poor.

DIARY OF A BIPOLAR EXPLORER

June 2017: Day of Rage

I swelter in the heat wave, a fan whirring on my desk. News is coming in of the mounting death toll at Grenfell Tower, with fears that uncountable migrants and asylum seekers may have been trapped in the building. Today is a "Day of Rage" in London. I wish I could go and join the protests, but aversion to travel in this heat (and, I'll admit it, fear of the violence that might be induced by aggressive police presence) keeps me at home. My own troubles seem very small by comparison with this shocking disaster. Like so many others all over the country I'm shaken to the core. I hide, taking my medication and trying to keep well – watching and waiting for the next swing in my mood.

June 2017: Tom Paine and Jeremy Corbyn

I've joined Momentum. I'm inspired by the way the Labour leadership is drawing on British socialist traditions, reaching back into its own history for strength and solidarity. I've written a poem about socialism in which I trace a continuity between two political heroes, Tom Paine and Jeremy Corbyn. I've dedicated this to Corbyn – and, encouraged by my mum and sister Gill, have posted it to him with a letter of appreciation.

Tom Paine's soul

for Jeremy Corbyn

The soul is not a king housed in an airy citadel
but a serf ploughing the broken land;
not aloof, but watchful and wary.

It is an axe to the rotten tree-trunk,
a spade to the stubborn soil, a hammer
beating a tune on an ancient anvil.

The soul is not ethereal, preparing for an afterlife,
but substantial and of this very world;
not silent but sentient, unruly.

It speaks in a voice that all can understand –
not beyond but through the body, like wind in the trees
or the steady wash of waves on sand.

The soul is not meek, but strong and fearless;
quick as mercury, fresh as raindrops,
bright as buds, and green as leaves unfurled.

It is work in progress – work that's never done.
There is no stand-off between spirit and matter;
they are not two entities, but one.

Diary of a Bipolar Explorer

July 2017: Facebook again

I vowed never again to go back on Facebook, but have now re-joined to keep an eye on the closed group that is an adjunct to the Hall Writers' Forum and to join another closed group that supports Corbyn. I belong to these groups and to a music group, but I'm not "friending" individuals. In this way I hope to control addictive tendencies. It's interesting to be for the most part a Facebook Lurker, only occasionally making posts. In the Corbyn group I can participate in collective enthusiasm and I have access to many news articles and videos that I wouldn't find for myself by trawling the internet. I feel much more in touch with the world, though haunted by an old familiar feeling of being a middle-class outsider. Occasionally I find myself in trouble. Responding to one of my clumsier posts, a member of the group commented, "this is class warfare, not a debate". I clearly betray my academic training even in brief exchanges. I imagine that my Oxford affiliations are off-putting to this community. Still, membership is a worthwhile eye-opener, and my addiction to social media is under control.

Chapter Seven: Adjustment

July 2017: A broken ankle

We were taking a walk at Nare Head in Cornwall when an invisible rut in the path caused me to twist my ankle suddenly. I fell forward, luckily onto grass; but because of my overweight body, the ankle fractured. Despite the pain I was able to walk back to the car – and I got through the rest of the day on paracetamol. But the ankle swelled up overnight and by morning it was clear I'd need to visit a hospital. At the Minor Injuries Clinic in St Austell we waited for hours in a hot room with lots of other people, all equally frazzled. (White walls without pictures. Hospital barrenness. Endless signage. Flickering strip-lights. Queues and delays. Overworked nurses. Children with injuries. Bins bearing the old familiar words "DOMESTIC WASTE ONLY".) I was x-rayed and they found that a small piece of my ankle had broken off. A kind and humorous nurse kept calling me "darling" in a broad Cornish accent. She fitted me with a big black support boot which reaches up to my knee and is held on by Velcro straps. She told me that this hideous boot matched my outfit. We had a good laugh and I hobbled around.

Back in Oxford it's grim being stuck indoors all day more or less immobile. There'll be at least three weeks of this trial to get through. We've cancelled our holiday trip to Ireland. I feel little pain now, just discomfort. I'm like a cat in hiding, licking its wounds. I curse my feeble and overweight body but my spirits aren't unduly lowered – which takes me by surprise. This must mean my mood is stable. The only thing to do is to make fun of myself and get on with whatever I can. I listen to music a lot and write. On the first night, trying to sleep with my leg in the big black boot, I was sleepless until 3.00 a.m, so I got up and composed this humorous curse to vent my anger. Many apologies to Sylvia Plath for stealing some ideas and words from her great poem "Daddy". I think my verses may be about more than my broken ankle…

The complaint of the sleepless broken-ankled boot-wearer

You do not do, black boot, you do not do.
I'd rather mend my foot with superglue
than go another day inside of you.
Your thick straps squeeze my leg and make me stew.
I cannot sleep at night because of you;
I cannot move, or sniff, or say achoo.

You do not do, black boot, you do not do.
I carry you around; you make me blue.

Chapter Seven: Adjustment

I'd rather that you were my daddy's shoe
(his big brown leather shoe, which I outgrew).
You may be shiny and you may be new
but you can't help me; you don't have a clue.

You do not do, black boot, you do not do.
I wouldn't say these words if they weren't true:
I'll kick you off, I'll flush you down the loo.
My bone will set itself. I don't need you.
So off you go, black boot – yes, that's right, shoo!
I'm through with you – I'm really truly through.

July 2017: Distraction

I'm chewing a lot of nicorettes; they keep my spirits up. I must be careful not to get addicted. I'm also checking in to Facebook more often, contributing more to the Corbyn group. One tiresome result of this is that I get interrupted in whatever I'm doing by recurrent bleeps on my mobile telling me a notification has come in. I wonder how Facebook enthusiasts keep this problem under control: constantly logging in fritters time and concentration. This could become a real menace. I'm reminded of TS Eliot's line, "distracted from distraction by distraction". Much that happens in social media makes me think of these words.

Diary of a Bipolar Explorer

July 2017: On the alert

The Big Black Boot is a real endurance test, especially on hot days. It's hard to feel positive. I've been so focused on struggling with my ankle that I've been forgetting to take medication for my mood disorder and I begin to feel really down. I'm also working into the nights and not getting much sleep. Is an episode brewing? I'm on the alert, and have gone back to the meds.

Last night I wrote this poem for the Corbyn group on Facebook – I'm preaching to the converted there, but at least writing a political poem takes me outside myself.

Austerity

The poor get poorer and their anger grows
as well-fed bankers load their heavy shelves
with solid gold in long and gleaming rows.
Shrugging off conscience, tax-evaders shirk
the obligations that the rest observe.
Crass politicians send the sick to work
then creep off to their summer hidey-holes:
their "strong and stable" system will not swerve,
self-serving policies their only goals.
Imbalance governs life. The young grow old

paying off debts; the lonely old live on
longer than they would wish or die of cold.
Good teachers leave their jobs. Fed-up and tired
by bureaucratic grind they turn instead
to Business – wretched, burnt-out, un-inspired.
Fat tycoons line silk pockets with the pounds
they've filched from those less greedy than themselves.
Celebrities grow rich while nurses make their rounds
at half the salary their work deserves.
More benefits are slashed and destitution looms;
the sad beleaguered strikers lose their nerves…
My list goes on and on: no end in sight
to exploitation, greed, abuse and blight.
While Tories are in power we must fight.

August 2017: My soul is…

Light in the morning between curtains that are never fully closed. The hum of early traffic on the London Road. The dry patch of earth under our pruned rosemary where stray cats used to hide. Pert daisies pushing up two days after the lawn's been mown. House-leeks clustering thickly by the kitchen door. Shadows under the absent cherry tree and the long grass beneath, where bulbs still grow. The horse-shoe shape made by diseased roots under our gnarled old pear-tree, where mushrooms appear like magic with their soft grey rubbery glow. My table by the window, piled high with books – many still to read. Bob Dylan's and Bruce Springsteen's songs all day... and all day, too, the soft coo-cooing of pigeons on house-tops and in trees; blackbirds carrying food to their young. Phone calls from Emma, lunches with Sandie, messages from long-lost friends, endless cups of weak tea. Poems everywhere, creative endeavour that will never end. The spirit of justice and equality embodied in Jeremy Corbyn at a turning-point which no-one can deny. Darkness late on a summer evening as the stars and moon and spirits shine. In this heat, the fan at night, whirring its cool undertone. *"Now in the grace of the world and always"* (Tom Paulin): things to do, and things that will remain undone.

August 2017: The end of a chapter

Perhaps because of a lull, I feel in the mood for summarising my findings by writing proverbs. What is it about a proverb that's so satisfying? Is it that the brevity convinces one of an irreducible wisdom? Is there something in the translation of personal experience into universal advice that's comforting? Nothing is axiomatic in life, yet proverbs seem to be medicinal. I've drawn up a list of my own proverbs below, which condense what I've learnt about Bipolar Disorder from many years of experiencing it.

Lucy's proverbs, aphorisms and home truths:

If you build your house over a disused well, learn to love glistening slug trails.

A taboo is like standing water. Flush it away and start anew.

Leave labelling to the bureaucrats and the bigots. There are more than enough of them.

The hornbeam will grow perfectly spherical if you don't plant it against a wall.

A stigma is like an ill-fitting coat; sooner bin it than let out the seams.

The insane are society's scapegoats and lepers.

Mental illness is invisible; this doesn't make it unreal.

Know your own mind. No one else can know it for you.

Balance is a pinpoint on a graph; normality a fiction outside the spectrum.

Diary of a Bipolar Explorer

A glow-worm's light may lead you on paths un-travelled.

A damaged friendship is like a bent picture-hook. No amount of hammering will give it purchase on the wall.

Beware of advice disguised as questions.

Hope is a needle threaded in the dark.

A good proverb is as nutritional as an egg.

Ten minutes chatting with a true friend are worth more than all the hours a professional can spare you.

The wise cat sleeps where the stone is warm.

What use is all your wisdom to a slug?

If your medicine cupboard begins to resemble an Aladdin's cave, lock its door and take up swimming.

Proverbs are formulaic, but there is no formula for wisdom.

Relax! Who hasn't at some point believed they were being watched by a spy camera?

If you think your boss is reading your private emails, it might as well be true.

One person's wise proverb is another's useless platitude.

218

Chapter Seven: Adjustment

The limits of empathy are not always apparent.

Only when you bite the apple do you find the worm.

Security cameras are not trained exclusively on one person.

Remember, you're only a tiny part of a much bigger problem.

Paranoia is a label for those who hate surveillance.

Guilt is a luxury.

For every prying gossip-monger there is someone who doesn't give a damn.

Keep your pleasures close and your addictions closer.

There is no Truth, only the various stories.

Emails are like postcards, open to view.

Privacy is a bourgeois illusion.

There is no outside.

When the mind is banished, where does the heart hide?

Better to lose your way ten times in a wood at night than to choose the quick way home and miss the owls.

DIARY OF A BIPOLAR EXPLORER

Away with qualifications!

Extremes mix.

Bananas are manna to the brain.

If you're feeling low, head for the fruit bowl, not the bottle.

Be patient. The wall may have an invisible tunnel.

Pause at the sign saying DOMESTIC WASTE ONLY.

An addict's resolutions are like patterns left by frost.

Be circumspect when "outing" your secrets.

A pigeon on the wing is worth three in a box, but it will shit everywhere.

As you crow, so may you creep.

The frost stays crisp in the tree's shadow.

When all else fails, listen to Bruce Springsteen's "Waitin' on a Sunny Day" and watch the official video.

"Everyone needs to love and be loved and keep going" (Kate Tempest, Glastonbury Festival 2017)

Aphorisms are the last refuge of an untidy mind.

Afterword:
Bipolarity and Life-Writing

As I bring this diary to completion it strikes me that my case history has raised questions about how Bipolar Disorder is approached in two different interlocking institutions – the family and the workplace. In both these contexts I've encountered difficulties in getting my condition understood. Individuals can be compassionate and in my experience they often are, especially when they happen to be friends. But *communities* are uncertain about how to deal adequately with disabilities. Mental illness is something that continues, even in 2017, to cause collective fear.

Since November of 2016 I've been receiving support from friends, from family, and from fellow-members of the Hall Writers' Forum for publication of this book. One HWF member said that his daughter recently graduated from an Oxford college where she experienced such "primitive" attitudes to mental health that this prompted her to enter a career in counselling. Another member, recently graduated, observed that there is ongoing unrest about the way in which Oxford handles mental illness. There's a sense on the Forum that outing my concerns in print will help others.

I could have written this as an angry book, pointing the finger at institutions which I feel let me down. But I have not done so. My mode in this diary is confessional, not accusatory. I recognise that my disability is mild compared with the suffering of many people: as an Oxford don I've led a privileged life in all material respects. Bereavement is common, everyone must deal with it as they reach a certain age – and retirement comes to us all. Anyone who is bipolar (or who reads the literature on bipolarity) will know that my experiences are typical, not extraordinary: families and workplaces understandably find it difficult to deal with disability and the mechanisms for doing so are fallible. I'm full of gratitude to individual friends and family members who now understand my illness and especially to the Hall Writers' Forum where I've found a supportive space in which to voice my concerns, express my feelings.

My anger at what I had to undergo as a consequence of psychosis in 2002 has only recently abated. This has happened through "outing" my illness and deciding to write this book – which of course meant I had to revisit the psychotic episode and involve my family in a reconstruction of what happened. I wrote most of the narrative in "Chapter One: The Showdown" without reference to their points of view. It was only by subsequently talking with my family and enabling their narratives to emerge (see the poems in Chapter Six) that I've come to terms with the way my psychosis terrified them and to feel less appalled by the indignity I was subjected to. The incompatibility of our narratives has taught me not to expect any coherent truth after so long a period of silence, but rather to see the ways in which each one of us has been trapped within our own subjective world of fear and grief. Turning our conversations into poems has brought me closer to my family. This has done a great deal to soften my memories of a traumatic experience. I no longer feel trepidation about crossing the threshold to my mum's flat.

Confession is a tricky medium to handle. "I should like in some way to make my soul transparent to the reader's eye," Rousseau wrote in his *Confessions*, "and for that purpose I am trying to present it from all points of view, to show it in all its lights, and to contrive that none of its movements shall escape his notice, so that he may

judge for himself of the principle that produced them."
A noble enough project, but he set the bar so high that
his protestations sound a hollow note, and we find him
anything but reliable:

> Since I have undertaken to reveal myself absolutely
> to the public, nothing about me must remain
> hidden or obscure. I must remain incessantly
> beneath his gaze, so that he may follow me in all
> the extravagances of my heart and into every least
> corner of my life. Indeed, he must never lose sight
> of me for a single instant, for if he finds the slightest
> gap in my story, the smallest hiatus, he may wonder
> what I was doing at that moment and accuse me of
> refusing to tell the whole truth.

My own aims have been, like his, transparency and candour.
But I've selected only fragments from a fifteen-year period
of my life, making no pretence to offer comprehensive
coverage. Have I slipped away, even more than Rousseau
did, in the gaps between these slivers of my case-history?

Most of my diary has been written retrospectively,
drawing on medical records, creative writings and e-mails
to achieve as much authenticity as possible. I've used a
mixture of narrative methods, switching from the past

Afterword: Bipolarity and Life-Writing

tense in Chapter One to the present tense (mostly) in the remaining chapters and in two places writing in the form of short story. "The Showdown" draws on notes which I wrote in the back of Susan Hill's *Strange Meeting* during the onset of my psychosis in 2002 and subsequently while sectioned at the psychiatric hospital in Leeds. The wording of the weekly questionnaires is accurate. In supplying 5 sample responses I've tried to build a balanced picture of my own pattern of illness, which has involved episodes of "mixed mood" with mania and depression coexisting. The consultations which follow each of the questionnaires are sometimes fictional reconstructions of conversations that have taken place with doctors and counsellors over a period of many years and sometimes an attempt to render internal questionings. Likewise, the personnel who appear in the book are fictionalised versions of real-life people. Real names have been retained for all family members.

Writing this book has not been cathartic. But it has enabled me to structure my case history and to see a pattern in the ups and downs of illness. There have been three key periods of crisis – around my dad's death in 2002, struggling with College in 2008-9, and negotiating the transition into retirement in November 2016 - spring 2017. I've explored some recurring themes in the lead-up to manic episodes,

225

and in the triggers that precipitate them. I've detected in myself a persistent obsession with death and a tendency to get involved in missions (small and large) that are fired by a sense of injustice or unfairness. The sibling rivalry which came to the fore during the psychotic episode in 2002 has sent its tremors across the years. A competitive streak in myself (without which I could not have succeeded professionally) is apparent, as is a recurring preoccupation with violence in and beyond the family. I've uncovered my ongoing difficulties with achieving balance and my intermittent failure to keep paranoid thoughts under control. I've also traced an emergence, in retirement, into political consciousness: this takes me outside the bubble of my personal preoccupations.

Friendship is one of the most important and sustaining things in everyone's life. For the bipolar patient it can be quite literally a lifeline. I haven't written much about my friendships. This has been out of respect for the privacy of people who may not wish to feature in my diary, not because of any lack of appreciation for their affection and support. My illness has sometimes put relationships under extreme strain. I've traced my difficulties within groups and communities – as well as in social media, where the word "friend" has arguably become debased.

AFTERWORD: BIPOLARITY AND LIFE-WRITING

("Oh my friends, there is no friend", wrote Aristotle.) To anyone suffering from Bipolar Disorder, I would say this: friendship is essential to sanity and balance. Take comfort in the people you really trust, and be reassured that this medical condition doesn't put you beyond the reach of love, though episodes of illness will sometimes test it.

Nature has emerged as an intermittently consoling presence. This diary has plotted my own story against the unfolding calendar of fifteen years. Each year, with its natural rhythms, has leant a kind of scaffolding to the narrative. I've allowed the seasons to peek through at times when I've been receptive to what they have to say. My book offers a kind of "back-story" to the poems of bereavement that appear in my collection, *Earth's Almanac*. Whereas the poems in that collection distil emotions, sublimating them into the structures and tropes of pastoral, my diary is a more humdrum record of moods as they unfold. The day-to-day entries show how my medical condition is always there, going through its own ups and downs no matter what else is happening. Poems have interrupted this diurnal pattern at moments of crisis to give their own different kind of testimony.

Throughout this book I have explored my love of poetry and my life as a creative writer. My diary has recorded my coming into being as a poet, bipolarity's role in stimulating creativity, and the struggle for authentic self-expression. "The truest poetry is the most feigning", Touchstone says to Audrey in Shakespeare's *As You Like It*. Is there something about verse (despite its artifice) that's more honest than writing a diary entry or an essay? Does a poem enable access to feelings and the unconscious in a way that prose can never quite achieve? Or is it the other way round – does verse involve more distance, through the discipline of metre and sometimes rhyme?

Robert Frost wrote that a poem is "a momentary stay against confusion". As both a poet and an academic I would say that verse provides a purer means of accessing memories and shaping thoughts than any other written medium. Verse proves valuable to me as someone with Bipolar Disorder because it enables a unique combination of self-expression and detachment. I find the challenge of using fixed verse forms to be effective in enabling me to stand back from the symptoms of my illness. I also find that the process of revising my poems calls on skills of attentiveness, judgement and self-criticism. Concentrating on the *crafting* of a poem is as good as drawing or gardening if one wants to achieve a balanced frame of mind. I find it even more effective than walking and diary-writing, though they too can be therapeutic.

Select Bibliography

Douglas Dunn, *Elegies* (Faber, 1985)

Peter Forbes, *We have come through: 100 Poems Celebrating Courage in Overcoming Depression and Trauma* (Bloodaxe, 2003)

Michel Foucault, *Madness and Civilization: A History of Insanity in the Age of Reason* (Psychology Press, 2001)

Lilias Fraser, ed., *Tools of the Trade: Poems for New Doctors* (Scottish Poetry Library, 2016)

Stephen Fry, *The Secret Life of the Manic Depressive* (Digital Classics, 2005)

Jay Griffiths, *Tristimania: A Diary of Manic Depression* (Hamish Hamilton/Penguin, 2016)

Mark Haddon, *Polar Bears* (Methuen Drama: *Modern Plays*, 2014)

Ted Hughes, *Birthday Letters* (Faber, 2002)

Kay Redfield Jamison, *Touched with Fire: Manic Depression and the Artistic Temperament* (Free Press, 1993)

--------------------------, *An Unquiet Mind: A Memoir of Moods and Madness* (Vintage Books, 1995)

-----------------------------, *Robert Lowell: Setting the River on Fire* (Alfred A Knopf, 2017)

Gwyneth Lewis, *Sunbathing in the Rain* (Harper Collins, 2005)

--------------------, *A Hospital Odyssey* (Bloodaxe Books, 2010)

Richard Mabey, *Nature Cure* (Chatto and Windus, 2005)

Lucy Newlyn, *Ginnel* (Oxford Poets, Carcanet, 2005)

------------------, *Earth's Almanac* (Enitharmon Press, 2015)

Sarah Owen and Amanda Saunders, *Bipolar Disorder – The Ultimate Guide* (Oneworld, 2008)

Sylvia Plath, *The Bell Jar* (Harper and Row, 1971)

Max Porter, *Grief is the Thing with Feathers* (Faber, 2015)

P. J. Rees & D. G. Williams *Principles of Clinical Medicine* (Hodder Arnold, 1995)

Oliver Sacks, *Musicophilia: Tales of Music and the Brain* (Vintage, 2008)

Ken Smith and Matthew Sweeney (eds) *Beyond Bedlam: poems written out of mental illness* (Anvil Press, 1997)

Sarah Wardle, *A Knowable World* (Bloodaxe Books, 2009)

Acknowledgements

In writing this book I've been helped by so many friends, family members and colleagues that I fear I may inadvertently miss out a name in thanking them.

My biggest debts are to my husband Martin, my daughter Emma, my sister Gill and my friend Sandie, all of whom have offered unflagging emotional support and encouragement. Gill has read the book in its various drafts, and I'm very grateful to her for her trenchant, insightful comments. Thanks also to my brother-in-law Chris Liddle, who suggested that I call this book 'Bipolar Explorer' (I have subsequently discovered that this phrase appears in Jay Griffiths' book, *Tristimania* -- and also that it's the name of a band!). I was very fortunate to have helpful conversations with my mother and my sister Kate at a crucial turning-point. Without my whole family's consent and enthusiasm I could not have gone ahead with publication.

A huge thank-you to the Hall Writers' Forum for their collective support, and especially to the following individual members of the Forum for advice, comment and feedback on the book as it has gone through various stages: Darrell Barnes, Nuzhat Bukhari, Tony Brignull, Jared Campbell, Tom Clucas, John-Mark Considine, Tony Hufton, Gerard Lally and Natasha Walker.

My step-daughter Fiona not only encouraged me to write the book, but acted as unofficial agent when I was seeking a publisher. Elsa Bell, former Head of Oxford University's Counselling Service, gave me expert professional feedback when the diary was in its final draft. Adrian Briggs, Fellow in Law at St Edmund Hall, also read it at the end – and offered timely reassurance.

Over the course of the last fifteen years I have come in contact with, and been helped by, many members of the medical profession. All of that experience has fed into this diary. I have also learned a great deal not just from the books which appear in the bibliography, but from years of teaching a life-writing course at Oxford alongside Hermione Lee. Last but not least, I'm grateful to my students for being there, for inspiring me with their work, and for putting up with me when I was not at my best.

There are many other friends whose affection I'm grateful for – especially Nicky Trott's. Thank you, one and all.